DIABETES

Foods, Supplements & Herbs

Isabel M. Rivero

COPYRIGHT & CREDITS

DIABETES. Foods, Supplements & Herbs.
Copyright ©2024 *by* Isabel M. Rivero
All rights reserved

Cover design: Desirée Mendoza M.
Photographs by Maja7777 and KenStock via Pixabay

I have written this book for my cousin, Rita M.M.

"I dedicate it to you with warm regards and heartfelt wishes.
I sincerely hope that the information and advice within
provide you the support you need to grow and improve each day."

Prologue: A Guide to Wellness

Dear Readers,

Welcome to this journey toward better health! Since I began sharing my knowledge and experience, my primary motivation has been to make a positive contribution to your lives. That's why, through these pages, I aim to offer valuable information and practical resources that can genuinely help you feel better.

In this book, every piece of advice and remedy has been thoughtfully chosen for its proven effectiveness and practicality in everyday life. You will discover not only medicinal plants, supplements, and accessible foods but also detailed medical insights into this health concern, along with additional tips and answers to the most frequently asked questions–providing you with a practical, comprehensive, and trustworthy guide.

My goal is for this work to be your valuable and practical companion–a resource where you can find tangible tools to support you on your journey toward a healthier, more fulfilling life. Knowing that this work has a positive impact brings me great joy and motivates me to keep going. While writing requires effort, time, and perseverance, the knowledge that my books make a meaningful difference in your lives is my greatest reward.

Because your experiences are my greatest source of inspiration, I would love for you to write to me and share your progress. Feel free to share your progress by writing directly to me at **isabelmriveror@gmail.com**. Your stories inspire me and truly make my efforts worthwhile.

I sincerely hope this practical guide becomes your indispensable pillar on your journey to better health and well-being. Thank you for allowing me to be part of your life.

With love,

Isabel

INTRODUCTION

On our journey towards achieving optimal health, it's crucial to recognize one fundamental truth: no single "miracle" solution –be it a medication, herb, supplement, or food–can fully resolve an illness on its own. Solely focusing on managing symptoms, while neglecting the deeper "root cause," not only delays true healing but also increases the likelihood of recurrence. Instead, addressing the underlying cause of the problem can lead to a gradual reduction in symptoms and support genuine, long-lasting recovery.

You may have experienced times when treatments or medications didn't seem to deliver the results you had hoped for. This often occurs because restoring health requires a holistic approach–one that goes beyond surface-level treatment to target the root cause of the issue. Effective healing involves more than just the right therapies; it must also encompass vital changes. A well-rounded plan should include improvements to diet (the cornerstone of cellular health), enhanced sleep quality, better stress management, and the cultivation of healthier daily lifestyle habits. Together, these elements strengthen the body's resilience, boost confidence in recovery, and reinforce its natural ability to heal.

This book takes you on a journey through this integrative approach to health and recovery. In the first chapter, we'll provide you with accessible, straightforward explanations of the main causes behind this particular illness. Additionally, we'll cover its key symptoms, variations, early warning signs, potential complications, practical advice to manage them, and the essential medical tests necessary for an accurate diagnosis. This foundation sets the stage for understanding your condition and equips you with the tools needed to address it effectively.

As the chapters unfold, you'll discover practical, evidence-based strategies designed to support your recovery. These include detailed dietary recommendations, easy-to-follow meal plans tailored to your needs, and natural approaches such as supplements and herbal remedies that support gradual, sustained improvement. The guidance provided is both flexible and adaptable, allowing you to choose what works best for your unique health journey.

For those seeking a clear roadmap, the chapter titled **"Suggested Practical Plan"** serves as a comprehensive guide. This section consolidates the most important elements of recovery into an actionable framework, while also pointing you toward additional chapters for deeper insights and tailored advice. By using this plan as your foundation, you'll gain clarity and confidence in navigating the steps toward healing.

It's worth stressing that the guidance in this book is not based on subjective opinions or anecdotal evidence. Rather, every recommendation is supported by scientific research and validated by credible studies. To further reassure you, we've included a comprehensive list of references and studies at the end of the book. This ensures you can trust the methods and feel secure when implementing these strategies into your life.

Through a blend of understanding, practical tips, and scientifically-backed solutions, this book aims to empower you as you work toward true recovery and lasting wellness.

DIABETES

Diabetes has accompanied humanity since ancient times. Diseases that we would now associate with diabetes were described as far back as in ancient Egyptian texts and Indian medical treatises, underscoring how deeply this condition is embedded in the history of our species. During the 19th century, significant scientific advancements in the study of metabolism and the endocrine system paved the way for the discovery of insulin in the early 20th century. This revolutionary breakthrough transformed diabetes from an almost inevitable death sentence into a manageable condition with proper treatment.

Diabetes is a disease that disrupts the way the body processes glucose, a fundamental sugar in our blood that serves as the primary energy source for our cells. To understand how diabetes impacts the body, it's helpful to first know how this process functions in a healthy individual. This foundation allows us to grasp what happens when something goes wrong.

When we eat, our food is broken down into essential nutrients, including carbohydrates, which are converted into glucose and absorbed into the bloodstream. Glucose acts as crucial "fuel" for our cells to function. However, for glucose to enter the cells, the body requires insulin, a vital hormone produced by the pancreas, an organ located behind the stomach. Under normal circumstances, after a meal, blood glucose levels rise, prompting the pancreas to release insulin. This hormone acts like a key, unlocking the "doors" of the cells and allowing glucose to enter, where it is used as energy. Once this process is complete, blood glucose levels return to normal.

In individuals with diabetes, this delicate balance is disrupted. Blood glucose levels remain elevated because the regulation mechanism fails to function properly. Depending on the type of diabetes, the causes and treatment approaches vary. In type 1 diabetes, the immune system, which is meant to protect the body from infections, mistakenly attacks the beta cells in the pancreas responsible for producing insulin. As a result, the body produces little to no insulin. Without insulin, glucose cannot enter the cells and accumulates in the bloodstream. People with this form of diabetes require daily insulin administration–whether through injections or an insulin pump–to regulate their blood glucose levels and ensure their survival.

Type 2 diabetes, on the other hand, emerges from a different mechanism. In this case, the body's cells develop resistance to insulin, meaning they don't respond effectively to the hormone. Additionally, the pancreas may be unable to produce enough insulin to compensate for this resistance. As a result, blood glucose levels rise. Although more commonly diagnosed in adults, type 2 diabetes is increasingly prevalent among younger individuals, driven by factors such as unbalanced diets, sedentary lifestyles, and rising obesity rates. Its treatment typically involves a combination of lifestyle changes, medication, and, in some cases, insulin therapy.

When glucose cannot enter the cells and remains in the bloodstream, various complications arise. Without the energy provided by glucose, the body's cells often suffer from extreme fatigue and weakness. In response, the body frequently resorts to burning fat as an alternative energy source. This process produces ketone bodies, such as acetone, acetoacetate, and beta-hydroxybutyrate. Under normal conditions, these substances are present at low levels. However, in people with diabetes–particularly when they do not receive sufficient insulin –this process can go into overdrive, leading to a dangerous condition known as diabetic ketoacidosis (DKA).

Diabetic ketoacidosis is a severe and potentially life-threatening complication that most commonly occurs in individuals with type 1 diabetes, though it can also arise in rare cases of type 2 diabetes. DKA occurs when blood glucose levels remain elevated for prolonged periods due to a lack of insulin, leading to an accumulation of ketone bodies that increase the acidity of the blood. This drop in pH can result in severe complications if not treated promptly.

This imbalance between insulin and glucose can significantly affect both short-term health and long-term well-being. Nevertheless, it is important to remember that you are not alone in this journey. With proper management and a strong understanding of the condition, serious complications can be prevented, and it is possible to maintain a good quality of life. The first essential step is to understand how diabetes affects your body. This knowledge empowers you to take control of your health and make informed decisions to protect your well-being.

This book has been designed as a comprehensive guide and ongoing source of support as you navigate this journey. Inside, you will find key information presented in an accessible way to help you better understand your condition, along with practical advice for adopting healthy habits that make a real difference. Remember, having the right tools and accurate knowledge can be the catalyst for creating a healthier, more fulfilling future. You have the power to take control of your health, improve your well-being, and enhance your quality of life!

Types of Diabetes

Although diabetes is often discussed as if it were a single disease, the reality is that there are several distinct types, each with its own specific causes, pathophysiological mechanisms, and treatments. Understanding these differences is crucial for achieving an accurate diagnosis and effective management of the condition, which can make a significant difference in the quality of life for those affected.

According to the most widely accepted classification, the primary types of diabetes include type 1 diabetes, type 2 diabetes, gestational diabetes, and several other less common specific types. Below, we will delve into each of these to better understand their unique characteristics and importance.

Type 1 Diabetes

Type 1 diabetes is a chronic autoimmune disease that accounts for approximately 5-10% of all cases of diabetes. In this condition, the immune system mistakenly attacks and destroys the beta cells of the pancreas, which are responsible for insulin production. Insulin is a vital hormone that regulates glucose metabolism in the blood, allowing glucose to enter the cells and be used as an energy source.

Medical treatment

Treatment of type 1 diabetes focuses on insulin administration, constant monitoring of glucose levels, and education on disease management.

Insulin therapy
‣ Rapid-acting insulin: Used before meals to control post-prandial glucose spikes (the glucose level in the blood that is measured after eating).
‣ Long-acting insulin provides a basal insulin level to control glucose between meals and at night.
‣ Insulin pumps: Devices that provide continuous insulin delivery, improving glycemic control.

Glucose monitoring
Continuous glucose monitors (CGM): They provide a detailed view of glucose fluctuations throughout the day.
Capillary glucose measurements: Allow adjustments in the daily treatment.

Type 2 Diabetes

Type 2 diabetes is a metabolic disease characterized by chronic hyperglycemia resulting from insulin resistance and progressive dysfunction of the pancreas's beta cells. It is the most common form of diabetes, accounting for approximately 90-95% of all cases worldwide. Unlike type 1 diabetes, it is not an autoimmune disease, and its development is strongly influenced by genetic and, above all, dietary and lifestyle factors.

Type 2 diabetes develops gradually and results from the body's inability to use insulin effectively (insulin resistance) and a relative decrease in the pancreas's insulin production.

Medical treatment

Management of type 2 diabetes focuses on improving insulin sensitivity and controlling blood glucose levels through dietary and lifestyle changes, medications, and, in some cases, insulin.

Dietary and lifestyle changes
▸ Diet: A balanced diet, rich in fiber and lean proteins and low in refined carbohydrates, simple sugars, and saturated fats, is fundamental.
▸ Exercise: Regular physical activity improves insulin sensitivity and aids in weight control.
▸ Weight loss: Even a modest reduction in body weight can significantly improve glycemic control.

Medications
▸ Metformin: It is usually the first drug prescribed, as it improves insulin sensitivity and reduces hepatic glucose production.
▸ SGLT2 inhibitors: Help reduce glucose levels by increasing its excretion through urine.
▸ GLP-1 agonists: Improve insulin secretion and reduce appetite.
▸ Sulfonylureas: Stimulate insulin release from the pancreas.
▸ Insulin: In cases where other treatments are insufficient, insulin may be necessary to control blood glucose.

Gestational Diabetes

Gestational diabetes is a type of diabetes that is first diagnosed during pregnancy in women who did not have diabetes before they became pregnant. This condition affects how the body's cells use glucose (sugar), leading to high blood glucose levels that can affect both mother and baby.

Treatment

The goal of treatment is to maintain blood glucose levels within a healthy range to protect the mother and baby. Management strategies include:

▸ Healthy eating: Following a balanced eating plan and controlling the intake of carbohydrates and sugars is crucial.
▸ Regular exercise: Moderate physical activity can help control glucose levels.
▸ Glucose monitoring: Monitor blood glucose regularly to ensure it remains within the target range.
▸ Medications: Insulin or oral medications may be necessary if dietary changes and exercise are insufficient.

Other Specific Types of Diabetes

In addition to gestational diabetes and the more well-known types of diabetes, such as type 1 and type 2 diabetes, other specific types of diabetes are less common but equally important to understand. Here are some of them:

Monogenic Diabetes

Monogenic diabetes is a rare type resulting from mutations in a single gene. Unlike type 1 and type 2 diabetes, it is not caused by environmental or lifestyle factors but by a genetic alteration that affects the body's ability to produce or use insulin properly. The most common types are MODY (Maturity Onset Diabetes of the Young) and neonatal diabetes.

Type 3C Diabetes

Also known as pancreatogenic diabetes, type 3c diabetes is a form of diabetes that results from dysfunction of the exocrine pancreas. This dysfunction may be caused by chronic pancreatitis, pancreatic surgery, pancreatic cancer, or cystic fibrosis, and it leads to decreased production of insulin and digestive enzymes.

Latent Autoimmune Adult-Onset Diabetes (LADA)

LADA is an autoimmune form of diabetes that develops in adults. Although it shares characteristics with type 1 diabetes (autoimmune destruction of the pancreas's beta cells), its progression is slower, and it is often initially confused with type 2 diabetes.

Drug or Chemical-Induced Diabetes

Certain medications or exposure to chemicals that affect glucose regulation in the body can cause this form of diabetes. Drugs that can cause this type of diabetes include glucocorticoids, some chemotherapeutic agents, and specific immunosuppressants.

Symptoms of the Different Types of Diabetes

Here, we will examine the key symptoms associated with each type of diabetes. Identifying these symptoms early is essential for obtaining a timely diagnosis and appropriate treatment, which can help prevent future complications and significantly improve quality of life. Let's take a closer look at the most common signs for each type of diabetes:

Type 1 Diabetes

Symptoms usually appear suddenly and may include:

‣ Increased thirst: Continuous sensation of thirst that is not easily relieved.
‣ Increased urge to urinate: Urgency to urinate frequently, especially at night.
‣ Extreme hunger: Constant feeling of hunger, even after eating.
‣ Involuntary weight loss: Weight loss despite an increase in food intake.
‣ Fatigue: A feeling of extreme tiredness and weakness.
‣ Blurred vision: Difficulty in focusing vision.

Type 2 Diabetes

Symptoms may be less evident at first and typically include:

‣ Increased thirst and need to urinate: Similar to the symptoms of type 1 diabetes.
‣ Excessive hunger: Persistent feeling of hunger.
‣ Fatigue: Tiredness and lack of energy.
‣ Blurred vision: Difficulties in seeing clearly.
‣ Frequent infections: Recurrent infections, especially of the skin and gums.
‣ Slow-healing wounds: Cuts and bruises take longer to heal.
‣ Darkening of the skin: Areas of dark skin, usually in the armpits and neck, known as acanthosis nigricans.

Gestational Diabetes

Gestational diabetes occurs during pregnancy and may have no apparent symptoms. However, some women may experience:

‣ Increased thirst and urinary frequency: Similar to other types of diabetes.
‣ Fatigue: Sensation of constant tiredness.

‣ Nausea: Some women may experience nausea, although this may also be related to the pregnancy itself.

Monogenic Diabetes

Symptoms of monogenic diabetes may vary depending on the specific type, but generally include:

‣ Excessive thirst (polydipsia).
‣ Frequent urination (polyuria).
‣ Unexplained weight loss.
‣ Fatigue.
‣ In some types, such as MODY, symptoms may be milder and are diagnosed incidentally during routine blood tests.

Type 3C Diabetes

Symptoms of type 3c diabetes may include:

‣ Classic symptoms of diabetes include excessive thirst and frequent urination.
‣ Weight loss.
‣ Abdominal pain or difficulty digesting due to exocrine pancreatic insufficiency.
‣ Malnutrition or vitamin deficiency due to malabsorption of nutrients.

Latent Autoimmune Diabetes of the Adult (LADA)

Symptoms of LADA may initially be similar to those of type 2 diabetes but progress to:

‣ Increased thirst and urination.
‣ Fatigue.
‣ Weight loss.
‣ Disease progression may be slower, and there may be an initial response to typical type 2 diabetes treatments before insulin is needed.

Drug or Chemical-Induced Diabetes

Symptoms are similar to those of other types of diabetes and include:

- Excessive thirst and frequent urination.
- Fatigue.
- Blurred vision.
- Weight loss.
- These symptoms may appear after starting a new medication or exposure to certain chemicals.

It is essential to keep in mind that, although symptoms may be common among the different types of diabetes, the context in which they appear (such as the presence of other diseases or the use of certain medications) is crucial for a proper diagnosis.

Causes

Diabetes, although it manifests similarly across all types with elevated blood glucose levels, has diverse origins. The causes vary depending on the specific type of diabetes, involving genetic, autoimmune, hormonal, environmental, and lifestyle factors. Understanding these causes not only helps us gain a better insight into the disease but also enables us to identify potential risks and strategies for its proper prevention and management.

Below, we will explore the main underlying causes of each type of diabetes to better understand their differences and how they influence the development of this condition.

Type 1 Diabetes

Type 1 diabetes is an autoimmune disease. This means that the body's immune system, which usually fights infections, mistakenly attacks and destroys the insulin-producing beta cells in the pancreas. Although the exact cause of this autoimmune attack is not fully understood, it is believed to involve a combination of genetic and environmental factors, such as the following:

- Genetics: Certain major histocompatibility complex (MHC) genotypes predispose to type 1 diabetes. These genotypes affect the way the immune system recognizes beta cells.
- Environmental factors: Various factors, such as viral infections (e.g., enteroviruses) and possibly exposure to certain

chemicals, can trigger the onset of the immune response.
‣ Autoimmune process: Autoreactive T cells attack beta cells, gradually decreasing the pancreas's ability to produce insulin.

Type 1 diabetes develops when the immune system mistakenly attacks the pancreas's beta cells. The destruction of these beta cells leads to an absolute insulin deficiency, resulting in increased blood glucose (hyperglycemia).

Type 2 Diabetes

Type 2 diabetes occurs when the body becomes insulin resistant or when the pancreas does not produce enough insulin to maintain normal blood glucose levels. The exact causes are not fully understood, but several factors contribute to the development of the disease:

‣ Genetic factors: Genetic predisposition plays a role in developing insulin resistance. People with a family history of diabetes are at increased risk.
‣ Environmental and lifestyle factors:
‣ Unhealthy diet: High in calories, saturated fats, refined carbohydrates and sugars, increases insulin resistance.
‣ Overweight and obesity: Visceral fat accumulation is significantly associated with insulin resistance.
‣ Sedentary lifestyle: Lack of physical activity contributes to decreased insulin sensitivity.

Over time, the pancreas's beta cells strive to compensate for insulin resistance by producing more insulin. However, this compensatory production is unsustainable in the long term, leading to beta cell dysfunction and eventual exhaustion.

Gestational Diabetes

Gestational diabetes occurs when a pregnant woman's body cannot produce enough insulin to meet the extra needs during pregnancy. This may be due to:

‣ Maternal age (over 25 years old).
‣ Pregnancy hormones: The placenta produces hormones that can lead to insulin resistance during pregnancy.

‣ Excess weight: Being overweight or obese before pregnancy increases the risk.

‣ Genetic factors: A family history of diabetes may increase the risk.

‣ Gestational diabetes in a previous pregnancy.

‣ Ethnicity (higher prevalence in African American, Hispanic, Native American, and Asian women).

Monogenic Diabetes

Monogenic diabetes is caused by mutations in a single gene that affects insulin production or function. These mutations can be inherited from a parent or arise spontaneously. Some of the genes involved are HNF1A, HNF4A, and GCK.

The specific genetic alteration determines the type and severity of monogenic diabetes.

Type 3C Diabetes

Type 3c diabetes develops due to damage or disease of the exocrine pancreas, which can be caused by chronic pancreatitis, pancreatic surgery, pancreatic cancer, or cystic fibrosis. Any damage to the pancreas that affects its ability to produce insulin can increase the risk of developing type 3c diabetes.

This damage affects the ability of the pancreas to produce insulin and digestive enzymes.

Latent Autoimmune Diabetes of the Adult (LADA)

LADA is caused by an autoimmune process in which the immune system attacks and destroys the beta cells of the pancreas that produce insulin. Unlike type 1 diabetes, this destruction is slower. Genetic and environmental factors, such as viral infections, may play a role in initiating this autoimmune response.

Although it presents in adulthood, individuals with LADA often have autoimmune markers similar to those of type 1 diabetes.

Drug or Chemical-Induced Diabetes

This type of diabetes is caused by prolonged or high-dose use of certain medications or exposure to chemicals that alter glucose metabolism. Some drugs involved include antipsychotics, glucocorticoids, chemotherapeutic agents, and immunosuppressants.

Exposure to certain chemicals or toxins may also contribute to impaired glucose regulation.

Possible Long-Term Complications

This section is designed to offer clear guidance and effectively highlight potential risks, with an emphasis on prevention. By doing so, you can take proactive steps to safeguard your well-being and minimize the likelihood of complications.

Poorly managed diabetes can trigger a range of serious complications that, over time, can affect multiple organs and systems throughout the body. These complications often develop gradually and can greatly diminish quality of life, highlighting the critical need for consistent and effective disease management.

In this section, we will delve into the most common complications associated with diabetes, with the goal of promoting awareness and fostering strategies for prevention and effective management to reduce their long-term impact.

Type 1 Diabetes

Type 1 diabetes, a chronic disease that usually develops in childhood or adolescence, requires careful management throughout life to minimize the risk of complications. Long-term complications are primarily the result of elevated blood glucose levels (hyperglycemia) over prolonged periods. Some of the more common complications are listed below:

▸ **Cardiovascular diseases:**
People with type 1 diabetes have a significantly increased risk of developing cardiovascular disease, including coronary heart disease, heart attack, and stroke. This is because hyperglycemia can damage the walls of blood vessels, making them more susceptible to plaque buildup and hardening (atherosclerosis).

‣ Diabetic nephropathy:

Type 1 diabetes can cause damage to the small blood vessels in the kidneys, affecting their ability to filter wastes from the blood. Over time, this can lead to chronic kidney disease or kidney failure. Close control of glucose and blood pressure is crucial to reduce nephropathy risk.

‣ Diabetic neuropathy:

This complication involves nerve damage. Peripheral neuropathy, which mainly affects the legs and feet, can cause symptoms such as pain, tingling, and loss of sensation. Autonomic neuropathy, on the other hand, can affect the nerves that control involuntary functions, causing digestive problems, sexual dysfunction and bladder problems.

‣ Diabetic retinopathy:

Retinopathy is damage to the eye's blood vessels that can lead to vision loss. In people with type 1 diabetes, the risk of retinopathy increases with the duration of the disease and inadequate glucose control. In severe cases, it can lead to retinal detachment and blindness.

‣ Foot problems:

People with type 1 diabetes may develop foot problems due to a combination of neuropathy (which reduces sensation) and poor circulation. This can increase the risk of ulcers and infections that, if not adequately treated, can lead to amputation.

‣ Periodontal disease:

Type 1 diabetes may also increase the risk of developing gum and tooth problems due to increased susceptibility to infections and inflammation caused by chronic hyperglycemia.

‣ Dermatologic complications:

People with type 1 diabetes may experience skin disorders such as bacterial and fungal infections, itching, and poor wound healing.

Effective management of type 1 diabetes involves controlling blood glucose levels and regularly monitoring blood pressure, cholesterol and other health factors. Comprehensive management and early detection of complications can help prevent or delay their progression.

Type 2 Diabetes

Type 2 diabetes is the most common form of diabetes and usually develops in adulthood, although it is also increasing in children and adolescents due to dietary and lifestyle factors. As with type 1 diabetes, long-term complications arise mainly due to poorly controlled blood glucose levels. The most important complications are detailed here:

‣ Cardiovascular diseases:
People with type 2 diabetes are at elevated risk for heart disease, including coronary heart disease, heart attacks, and strokes. Hyperglycemia contributes to blood vessel damage and the development of atherosclerosis, while insulin resistance, hypertension, and dyslipidemia, commonly associated with type 2 diabetes, further increase this risk.

‣ Diabetic nephropathy:
Type 2 diabetes can lead to progressive kidney damage. High glucose levels damage the nephrons and filtering units of the kidney, resulting in chronic kidney disease. Early detection through kidney function tests and control of glucose and blood pressure are critical to prevent or delay this complication.

‣ Diabetic neuropathy:
This complication affects approximately 50% of people with type 2 diabetes. Peripheral neuropathy can cause pain, numbness, or loss of sensation, especially in the lower extremities, which increases the risk of injuries and ulcers. Autonomic neuropathy can cause digestive problems, sexual dysfunction and impaired bladder control.

‣ Diabetic retinopathy:
The risk of retinopathy increases with the duration of diabetes and poor glucose control. This condition can lead to decreased vision and, in severe cases, blindness. Regular eye examinations are critical for early detection and treatment.

‣ Foot problems:

The combination of poor circulation and neuropathy increases the risk of serious foot problems. Foot ulcers can quickly become infected and, if not adequately treated, can require amputation.

‣ Periodontal disease:

Type 2 diabetes is associated with an increased risk of gum disease, which can lead to tooth loss if left untreated. Hyperglycemia contributes to a more favorable environment for oral bacteria and chronic gum inflammation.

‣ Dermatologic complications:

People with type 2 diabetes may suffer from various skin conditions, including bacterial and fungal infections, itching, and poor wound healing.

‣ Cognitive complications:

Type 2 diabetes has also been associated with an increased risk of cognitive impairment and dementia. Chronic hyperglycemia, along with other cardiovascular risk factors, may contribute to cerebral vascular damage.

Management of type 2 diabetes focuses on controlling blood glucose, adopting a healthy lifestyle, and monitoring other risk factors such as blood pressure and cholesterol. Regular doctor visits and screening tests are essential for preventing and managing these complications.

Gestational Diabetes

Gestational diabetes is a type of diabetes that develops during pregnancy and usually disappears after delivery. The most common complications are listed below:

‣ Cesarean delivery:

Because of the risk of fetal macrosomia, mothers with gestational diabetes are more likely to need a cesarean section, which carries its own surgical and recovery risks.

‣ High blood pressure and preeclampsia:

Gestational diabetes increases the risk of developing high blood pressure during pregnancy, which can lead to severe conditions such as preeclampsia, which poses a danger to the life of both mother and baby.

▶ Risk of type 2 diabetes:
Women with gestational diabetes have a higher risk of developing type 2 diabetes later in life if they do not take care of their diet and lifestyle.

Monogenic Diabetes

Long-term complications can be similar to those of type 1 or type 2 diabetes, depending on glycemic control, and include:

▶ Cardiovascular disease.
▶ Neuropathy (nerve damage).
▶ Nephropathy (kidney damage).
▶ Retinopathy (eye damage).
▶ Complications in pregnancy are not adequately controlled, especially in cases such as monogenic gestational diabetes.

Type 3C Diabetes

Long-term complications may include:

▶ Vascular disease.
▶ Neuropathy.
▶ Nephropathy.
▶ Nutritional deficiencies are due to malabsorption of nutrients.
▶ Increased risk of additional pancreatic complications due to the underlying disease.

Latent Autoimmune Diabetes of the Adult (LADA)

Long-term complications are similar to those of type 1 diabetes, including:

▶ Cardiovascular disease.
▶ Neuropathy.
▶ Nephropathy.
▶ Retinopathy.
▶ Increased risk of additional autoimmune complications since LADA is an autoimmune disease.

Drug or Chemical-Induced Diabetes

Possible long-term complications depend on glucose control and may include:

‣ Cardiovascular disease.
‣ Neuropathy.
‣ Nephropathy.
‣ Retinopathy.
‣ Possible additional complications related to the long-term effects of the drug or chemical that induced the diabetes.

In conclusion, all forms of diabetes, when not properly managed, can result in chronic complications that profoundly impact overall health. Achieving and maintaining optimal blood glucose levels, regularly monitoring other risk factors, adhering to a balanced diet, and embracing a healthy lifestyle are crucial steps to minimize the risk of these complications and to ensure an improved quality of life over the long term.

Symptoms Reduction and Prevention

Diabetes, in any of its forms, represents a significant health challenge, but effective management can make a profound difference. With the right strategies and an evidence-based approach, it is possible not only to manage symptoms effectively but also to prevent long-term complications.

This section will focus on exploring actionable measures that support comprehensive diabetes management, aiming to enhance quality of life, minimize associated risks, and promote sustained well-being.

Type 1 Diabetes

Diminished symptoms:
‣ Balanced nutrition: meal planning that balances carbohydrates with protein and healthy fats. We will discuss this in the "Food" chapter.
‣ Regular exercise: Regular physical activity helps us use glucose more effectively.
‣ Tight glucose control: Appropriate use of insulin is vital for maintaining blood glucose levels within a target range.

‣ Frequent monitoring: Use blood glucose meters or continuous monitoring systems to adjust insulin doses and carbohydrate intake.

‣ Education and self-care: Understanding the effects of diet, exercise, and other factors on glucose control.

Prevention:

Currently, there are no proven methods to prevent type 1 diabetes, as it is an autoimmune disease with a significant genetic component. However, early detection and proper management can significantly improve the prognosis.

Type 2 Diabetes

Diminished symptoms:

‣ Healthy eating: Focus on whole foods rich in fiber and low in refined sugars and saturated fats. We will discuss this in the "Food" chapter.

‣ Lifestyle improvements: Increased physical activity and weight loss can improve insulin sensitivity.

‣ Medications: Use oral or injectable drugs to help control glucose levels when lifestyle modifications are insufficient.

‣ Regular monitoring: Blood glucose levels are monitored to adjust treatment as needed.

Prevention:

Prevention of type 2 diabetes is possible, especially in people at high risk, through dietary and lifestyle modifications. Prevention focuses primarily on the following:

‣ Adopt a balanced diet: Eat a diet rich in fruits, vegetables, whole grains, and low in saturated fats and refined sugars, among others (Read chapter "Nutrition").

‣ Maintaining a healthy weight: Weight loss and body mass index (BMI) within healthy ranges are critical.

‣ Increase physical activity: You should get at least 150 minutes of moderate exercise per week, such as walking, swimming, or cycling.

‣ Manage stress: Stress management through relaxation techniques, meditation, or yoga can help maintain hormonal balance and reduce the risk of developing diabetes.

‣ Regular monitoring of glucose and other markers: For those

problem under medical supervision.
‣ Regular blood glucose monitoring.
‣ Healthy diet. This will be discussed in the chapter "Nutrition".
‣ Regular exercise.

Prevention:
‣ Prudent and supervised use of medications that could induce diabetes.
‣ Regular consultation with health professionals to monitor the side effects of oncological or pharmacological treatments.

Additional Tips

In addition to the recommendations outlined in the chapter "Suggested Practical Plan", there are other complementary strategies that can be extremely valuable for effectively managing this condition. Below, we present a series of additional tips that are applicable to all types of diabetes to enhance management and improve overall quality of life.

‣ **Foot care**
People with diabetes are more prone to foot problems due to neuropathy and poor circulation.
Tip: Inspect your feet daily, moisturize the skin, wear appropriate footwear, and see a podiatrist regularly.

‣ **Smoking cessation and moderate alcohol consumption**
Smoking and excessive alcohol consumption can exacerbate diabetes complications.
Tip: If you smoke, seek help to quit. Limit alcohol consumption and always check your glucose levels before drinking.

‣ **Monitoring of other health parameters**
Diabetes can affect multiple aspects of health.
Tip: Regularly check blood pressure, cholesterol levels and kidney function, and perform annual eye exams.

‣ **Creation of a support network**
Having the support of family, friends, and health professionals is crucial.

Tip: Join support groups for people with diabetes, share your experiences, and learn from others' experiences.

‣ **Adequate hydration**
Staying well-hydrated is essential for optimal body function.
Tip: Drink enough water throughout the day and limit consumption of sugary drinks. Adequate hydration also helps to maintain stable glucose levels. The "Juices & Smoothies" chapter will discuss this in detail.

‣ **Emergency Preparedness**
Being prepared for emergencies is vital to the safety of people with diabetes.
Tip: Always carry medical identification that indicates you have diabetes. In case of hypoglycemia, keep a supply of fast-acting glucose, such as glucose tablets or candy.

‣ **Education of family and friends**
Having an informed support network can make a big difference in managing diabetes.
Tip: Educate your loved ones about diabetes and how they can help you in an emergency, especially in recognizing symptoms of hypoglycemia or hyperglycemia.

‣ **Regular medical visits**
Periodic medical check-ups are essential to monitor progress and adjust treatment.
Tip: Schedule regular consultations with your physician, endocrinologist and other specialists as needed, and discuss any changes in your symptoms or lifestyle.

‣ **Use of technology**
Technology can be a powerful tool in diabetes management.
Tip: Consider using continuous glucose monitors (CGMs), insulin pumps, and mobile apps to monitor your glucose levels and manage your diet and exercise. Consult with your doctor about which technology is right for you.

‣ **Prevention of long-term complications**
Poorly controlled diabetes can lead to serious complications over time.

Tip: Besides glucose control, maintain healthy blood pressure and cholesterol levels.

‣ Dental care

People with diabetes have an increased risk of dental and gum problems.

Tip: Brush your teeth at least twice a day, floss regularly, and visit the dentist for cleanings and checkups at least twice a year.

‣ Adaptation to life changes

Living with diabetes may require adjustments at different stages of life.

Tip: Be flexible and open to changing your routines and treatment plans as your life changes, such as hormonal changes, starting new activities, or aging.

‣ Positive approach and proactive attitude

Maintaining a positive attitude can significantly influence diabetes management.

Tip: Cultivate a positive mindset and seek emotional support if you feel overwhelmed. Remember that diabetes is manageable and that, with proper care, you can live a full and active life.

Diagnostic Medical Tests

A precise and timely diagnosis of diabetes is essential for implementing appropriate treatment and preventing potential long-term complications. Healthcare professionals have a range of diagnostic tests available to identify diabetes and monitor blood glucose levels. Below, we outline the most common tests and their roles in managing this condition effectively.

1. Fasting Plasma Glucose (FPG)

This test measures glucose levels in the blood after a fast of at least 8 hours. It is an essential and commonly used test for the initial diagnosis of diabetes.

Diagnostic values:
‣ Normal: Less than 100 mg/dL.
‣ Prediabetes: 100-125 mg/dL.
‣ Diabetes: 126 mg/dL or more on two separate occasions.

2. Oral Glucose Tolerance Test (OGTT)

This test evaluates the body's response to an ingested glucose load. Blood glucose is measured by fasting for 2 hours after drinking a specific sugar solution. It is handy for diagnosing diabetes in cases of prediabetes or gestational diabetes.

Diagnostic values:
- Normal: Less than 140 mg/dL at 2 hours.
- Prediabetes: 140-199 mg/dL at 2 hours.
- Diabetes: 200 mg/dL or more at 2 hours.

3. Hemoglobin A1c (HbA1c)

This test measures average blood glucose levels over the past 2-3 months by assessing the percentage of glucose-coated hemoglobin. It is a key tool for diagnosing and monitoring long-term diabetes control.

Diagnostic values:
- Standard: Less than 5.7%.
- Prediabetes: 5.7%-6.4%.
- Diabetes: 6.5% or more.

4. Random plasma glucose

Blood glucose can be measured at any time of the day, regardless of when the last meal was eaten. This is useful for rapid diagnosis in the presence of acute symptoms.

Diagnostic values:
- Diabetes: 200 mg/dL or more, along with classic symptoms of hyperglycemia (such as excessive thirst, frequent urination, and unexplained weight loss).

5. Additional tests for specific types of diabetes
- Autoantibodies (Type 1 diabetes): Tests for autoantibodies such as GAD, IA-2, and ICA can help distinguish autoimmune type 1 diabetes from type 2 diabetes.
- Genetic Evaluation (Monogenic Diabetes): Genetic testing can identify specific mutations in suspected cases of monogenic diabetes.
- Insulinoma or C-Peptide Testing: Assessments of insulin and C-peptide levels can help understand endogenous insulin

production.

6. Additional monitoring

‣ Lipid Profile and Renal Function: Tests to monitor lipid profile and renal function are essential in the comprehensive management of diabetes.
‣ Blood Pressure and Eye Exams: Regular blood pressure evaluations and fundus exams help prevent and manage complications.

Diagnosing diabetes involves the use of specific tests to ensure accuracy and develop a treatment plan tailored to each individual's needs. Every test serves a vital purpose and is selected based on the clinical context and the unique circumstances of each person. A comprehensive approach that integrates these tests with a thorough assessment of medical history and symptoms is crucial for effective and personalized diabetes management, supporting improved long-term health outcomes.

Warning Signs

The onset of certain warning signs in individuals with diabetes may signal the need for immediate medical attention. These symptoms, which must not be overlooked, include:

‣ **Severe hypoglycemia**: If a person with diabetes experiences symptoms of severe hypoglycemia, such as confusion, loss of consciousness, or seizures, it is crucial to seek immediate medical attention. Severe hypoglycemia can be dangerous if not treated quickly.

‣ **Diabetic ketoacidosis (DKA)** is a life-threatening condition caused by the body's production of high levels of acids called ketones in the blood. Symptoms include extreme thirst, frequent urination, nausea, vomiting, abdominal pain, weakness, fruity-smelling breath and confusion.

‣ **Hyperosmolar hyperglycemic non-ketotic syndrome**: This syndrome is characterized by extremely high blood glucose levels without ketones. Symptoms may include severe dehydration, confusion, weakness and coma.

▸ **Infections**: People with diabetes are more susceptible to infections, especially in the skin, feet, kidneys and bladder. If an infection seems to worsen rapidly, it is vital to seek medical attention.

▸ **Vision problems**: Sudden vision changes may indicate diabetes-related complications, such as diabetic retinopathy or macular edema. If you experience sudden visual changes, consult a physician immediately.

▸ **Chest pain or shortness of breath**: These may be signs of a heart attack or other cardiovascular complications that are more common in people with diabetes.

▸ **Non-healing wounds**: Wounds or ulcers that do not heal properly, especially on the feet, can lead to serious infections and require urgent medical attention.

Wounds on the Sole of the Foot and Diabetic Foot

In people with diabetes, ulcers or wounds often develop on the sole of the foot, particularly in areas exposed to increased pressure or friction. Commonly affected areas include the space between the first and second toes or the nearby metatarsal region. These issues arise from several factors related to the condition, including:

- **Diabetic Neuropathy**: Reduced sensitivity in the feet prevents individuals from noticing injuries, calluses, or friction, allowing wounds to develop unnoticed and untreated in time.

- **Peripheral Vascular Disease**: Poor blood flow slows down the healing process and increases the risk of infections.

- **Pressure or Foot Deformities**: Conditions such as high arches, bunions, or other deformities can concentrate pressure on specific areas, increasing the likelihood of injuries.

‣ Complications of These Wounds

If not detected and treated in time, these wounds can progress to serious complications, including:

- **Diabetic Ulcers**: A wound left untreated can develop into an infected ulcer, significantly increasing the risk of deep infections.

- **Advanced Infections**: Wounds can become severely infected, affecting bones and deep tissues. In complicated cases, this may lead to osteomyelitis or gangrene.

- **Risk of Amputation**: In advanced stages, if infections or ulcers are not controlled, amputations may be required to prevent the spread of infection.

‣ Prevention and Care

To reduce the risk of developing these wounds and their complications, it is essential to:

- **Daily Inspection**: Check your feet daily, especially between the toes, for redness, cuts, blisters, or any warning signs.

- **Footwear Care**: Wear comfortable, well-fitting shoes, avoiding footwear that causes pressure points.

- **Proper Hygiene**: Keep your feet clean and dry, paying special attention to the spaces between your toes.

- **Early Medical Attention**: Seek immediate medical care for any wounds or signs of infection to prevent more severe complications.

Preventive care and strict blood sugar control play a crucial role in protecting against these diabetic foot complications. Regular evaluations by a specialist are also key!

FREQUENTLY ASKED QUESTIONS

Navigating the intricate world of health can feel overwhelming, especially when faced with a diagnosis that affects both physical and emotional well-being. In such moments, many questions naturally arise: What does this mean for me? What options are available? How will my daily life change? Uncertainty and concern are common. Here, you'll discover practical and direct insights to help you make confident, informed choices.

This chapter was created to offer support and provide clear, straightforward tools to guide you through this journey. In today's era of abundant information, distinguishing reliable knowledge from content that might cause confusion is vital. With this in mind, I've compiled evidence-based guidance to help you navigate uncertainty with greater clarity.

The format of this resource prioritizes accessibility, addressing common concerns faced by individuals and families alike. Each explanation is concise, clear, and aimed at empowering you to make decisions that align with your overall well-being.

While the material here is designed to assist, it is not a substitute for personalized advice from healthcare professionals. Consulting your doctor for guidance tailored to your specific needs remains essential, especially to address challenges unique to your situation.

Through these pages, my goal is to foster calm, confidence, and reassurance so that you can approach your circumstances with strength and resolve. I hope this resource inspires you and provides the valuable tools necessary to manage your health effectively and confidently.

134 FAQs about Diabetes

1. What is diabetes?

Diabetes is a chronic disease that affects the body's ability to regulate blood glucose levels. The body either does not produce enough insulin or does not use it effectively.

2. What are the main types of diabetes?

There are three main types: type 1 diabetes, type 2 diabetes and gestational diabetes. Type 1 is an autoimmune disease, type 2 is related to lifestyle and genetic factors, and gestational diabetes occurs during pregnancy.

3. What are the common symptoms of diabetes?

Symptoms include excessive thirst, frequent urination, extreme hunger, unexplained weight loss, fatigue and blurred vision.

4. How is diabetes diagnosed?

Diabetes is diagnosed through blood tests that measure glucose levels: the fasting glucose test, the glucose tolerance test and the hemoglobin A1c test.

5. What is the difference between type 1 and type 2 diabetes?

Type 1 diabetes is an autoimmune condition in which the immune system destroys insulin-producing cells in the pancreas. Type 2 diabetes is more common and develops when the body becomes insulin-resistant or does not produce enough insulin.

6. Is it possible to prevent type 2 diabetes?

Yes, it is possible to prevent or delay type 2 diabetes through lifestyle changes, such as following a healthy diet, maintaining an adequate weight, controlling stress, avoiding smoking, avoiding excessive alcohol consumption, and regular physical activity.

7. What complications can arise from diabetes?

Complications can include heart disease, kidney damage, eye damage, neuropathy (nerve damage), and foot problems that can lead to amputations, among others.

8. How is diabetes treated?

Diabetes treatment may include medications (such as insulin or metformin), dietary changes, regular exercise, and frequent monitoring of blood glucose levels.

9. Can people with diabetes lead a normal life?

Yes, with proper disease management and by making lifestyle changes, people with diabetes can lead a full and healthy life.

10. What role does nutrition play in the management of diabetes?

Diet is crucial in managing diabetes. A balanced diet rich in fiber and low in sugars and saturated fats helps control blood glucose levels and maintain a healthy weight.

11. What diet is most advisable for people with diabetes?

A balanced diet with complex carbohydrates, fiber, lean proteins and healthy fats is recommended. Mediterranean and low-carbohydrate diets have also been shown to be beneficial in managing diabetes.

12. Is it possible to reverse diabetes?

Although diabetes cannot currently be "cured", some people can achieve remission of type 2 diabetes through significant weight loss and dietary and lifestyle changes.

13. What is hypoglycemia, and how is it managed?

Hypoglycemia is an abnormally low blood glucose level. It is managed by quickly consuming fast-acting carbohydrates, such as fruit juice or glucose tablets, and then eating a snack containing protein or complex carbohydrates.

14. What are the warning signs of low blood sugar (hypoglycemia)?

Symptoms of hypoglycemia include tremors, sweating, confusion, hunger, irritability, dizziness, and, in severe cases, loss of consciousness. It is crucial to treat it quickly by consuming fast-acting carbohydrates.

15. What is nocturnal hypoglycemia, and how can it be prevented?

Nocturnal hypoglycemia occurs when blood glucose levels drop too low during the night. It can be prevented by adjusting insulin dosage, eating a snack before bedtime, and monitoring glucose levels before bedtime.

16. What is inadvertent hypoglycemia, and how can it be managed?

Inadvertent hypoglycemia occurs when a person does not feel the symptoms of low blood glucose levels, which can be dangerous. Treatment adjustments and more frequent monitoring can manage it.

17. What is insulin resistance?

Insulin resistance is when the body's cells do not respond adequately to insulin, forcing the pancreas to produce more insulin to maintain normal blood glucose levels. It is a common precursor to type 2 diabetes.

18. How can insulin resistance be improved?

It can be improved through lifestyle changes such as healthy eating, regular exercise and weight loss.

19. What is gestational diabetes?

Gestational diabetes is a type of diabetes that develops during pregnancy. It affects how cells use glucose and can cause high blood sugar levels, affecting both mother and baby. It usually goes away after delivery, but it increases the risk of developing type 2 diabetes in the future for both mother and child.

20. How is gestational diabetes managed?

It is managed primarily with diet and exercise, but some women may need insulin or oral medications.

21. How is gestational diabetes diagnosed?

Glucose tolerance tests, which evaluate how the body handles sugar after ingesting a sugary drink, are performed during the second trimester of pregnancy to diagnose gestational diabetes.

22. Does diabetes affect mental health?

Yes, diabetes can affect mental health. The constant management of the disease can lead to stress, anxiety, and depression. Addressing these issues with psychological support and stress management strategies is essential.

23. What is the glycemic index, and why is it important?

The glycemic index (GI) measures how carbohydrate-containing foods affect blood glucose levels. Foods with a low GI are absorbed more slowly and are better at maintaining stable glucose levels.

24. What types of exercises are recommended for people with diabetes?

Aerobic exercises, such as walking, swimming, or cycling, and resistance exercises, such as weight lifting, are highly recommended.

25. Can aloe vera help in the management of diabetes?

Aloe vera has hypoglycemic properties and improves insulin sensitivity. However, it is essential to use it under medical supervision to avoid possible drug interactions.

26. What should family members of a person with diabetes know?

Family members should understand the signs of hypoglycemia and hyperglycemia, know how to act in an emergency, and support the person in managing nutrition and exercise.

27. What is ketosis, and how is it related to diabetes?

Ketosis is a metabolic process in which the body uses fat instead of glucose as energy. Uncontrolled ketosis can lead to diabetic ketoacidosis, a dangerous condition, in people with diabetes, especially those with type 1 diabetes.

28. What is diabetic ketoacidosis and its symptoms?

Diabetic ketoacidosis (DKA) is a serious complication of diabetes, most common in type 1 diabetes. It occurs when the body produces high levels of ketones due to a lack of insulin, leading to a dangerous imbalance of chemicals in the blood. Symptoms include nausea, vomiting, abdominal pain, rapid breathing or shortness of breath, and confusion. Diabetic ketoacidosis requires immediate medical attention.

29. How can diabetic ketoacidosis be prevented?
Diabetic ketoacidosis can be prevented with reasonable glucose control and immediate medical attention in case of warning symptoms.

30. How is diabetic ketoacidosis treated?
Treatment of diabetic ketoacidosis involves rehydration, electrolyte replacement and insulin administration.

31. How does diabetes affect oral and dental health?
People with diabetes are at increased risk for oral problems, such as infections, dry mouth and gum disease, due to reduced resistance to infection, decreased ability of the body to fight bacteria, and slow healing. Careful blood glucose control and good oral hygiene can help prevent these problems.

32. What is the metabolic syndrome and its relation to diabetes?
Metabolic syndrome is a group of conditions that occur together and increase the risk of heart disease, stroke and type 2 diabetes. These conditions include hypertension, high blood sugar levels, excess body fat around the waist, abnormal triglyceride levels, and low HDL cholesterol(the "good" cholesterol).

33. What impact does stress have on diabetes?
Stress can affect blood glucose levels by releasing hormones such as cortisol and adrenaline, which increase blood sugar. Managing stress is crucial to controlling diabetes.

34. How can stress be managed in people with diabetes?
Stress management is vital, as stress often negatively affects blood glucose control. Techniques such as meditation, regular exercise, mindfulness, deep breathing and psychological or social support can be helpful.

35. What is diabetic neuropathy?
Diabetic neuropathy is a type of nerve damage that can occur in people with diabetes. It mainly affects the nerves in the legs and feet and can cause symptoms such as pain, tingling, numbness, or loss of sensation.

36. What types of diabetic neuropathy are there?

Diabetic neuropathy is damage to the nerves. Types include peripheral, autonomic, proximal, and focal neuropathy, each affecting different body parts.

37. How does alcohol consumption affect people with diabetes?

Alcohol can affect blood sugar levels in several ways. In small amounts, it can cause a decrease in blood sugar, while in excess, it can raise it. People with diabetes should consume alcohol in moderation and always with food. It can interact with diabetes medications, so it should be consumed in moderation and under medical supervision.

38. What role do carbohydrates play in a person's diet with diabetes?

Carbohydrates directly affect blood glucose levels. Therefore, counting and controlling carbohydrate intake is essential to keep blood sugar within target ranges.

39. What is continuous glucose monitoring, and how does it work?

A continuous glucose monitoring (CGM) system measures glucose levels in interstitial fluid every few minutes using a sensor placed under the skin. It provides real-time information for better diabetes management.

40. How can diabetes affect pregnancy?

Diabetes during pregnancy can increase the risk of complications such as high blood pressure, premature delivery, and problems for the baby, such as increased fetal size.

41. How does diabetes affect the immune system?

Diabetes can weaken the immune system, increasing the risk of infections like urinary tract and skin infections. This is because high blood glucose levels can affect the function of immune cells.

42. What is dawn hyperglycemia, or the dawn phenomenon, in people with diabetes?

The dawn phenomenon is a natural rise in blood glucose levels in the early morning due to hormonal changes that prepare the body to wake up. It can be a challenge for people with diabetes to maintain control of their blood sugar upon awakening.

43. How can weight loss improve the control of type 2 diabetes?

Weight loss usually improves insulin sensitivity and lowers blood glucose levels. This also reduces the need for medication and lowers the risk of complications. Losing weight helps control and may reverse type 2 diabetes in some people.

44. What is a diabetic foot?

Diabetic foot refers to several problems that can affect the feet of people with diabetes, including ulcers, nerve damage to the feet, infections, and, in severe cases, amputations due to poor circulation and nerve damage.

45. Can diabetic foot be prevented?

Controlling blood sugar levels, practicing foot care, and visiting a podiatrist regularly can prevent diabetic foot pain.

46. Is diabetes hereditary?

There is a genetic component to diabetes, especially type 2 diabetes. However, lifestyle and environment play a crucial role in its development.

47. How important is regular blood pressure control in people with diabetes?

Controlling blood pressure is vital because hypertension can increase the risk of cardiovascular, renal, and ocular complications in people with diabetes.

48. How is sleep apnea related to diabetes?

Sleep apnea is more common in people with type 2 diabetes and can worsen blood sugar control. Treating sleep apnea can improve glucose levels and quality of life.

49. What is hemoglobin A1c, and what is its importance in diabetes?

Hemoglobin A1c is a test that measures average blood glucose levels over the past two to three months. It is a key tool for assessing long-term control of diabetes and for adjusting treatment. An A1c level below 7% is generally considered reasonable control for most adults with diabetes, although targets may vary from person to person.

50. Is intermittent fasting recommended for people with diabetes?

Intermittent fasting can be beneficial for some people with type 2 diabetes, helping to improve insulin sensitivity and lose weight. However, it is crucial to do it under medical supervision to avoid hypoglycemia or decompensation.

51. Are there supplements that can help control diabetes?

Some supplements, such as chromium, cinnamon and alpha-lipoic acid, have shown potential in scientific studies to improve insulin sensitivity and control blood sugar. However, it is essential to consult with a health professional before taking any supplements, as they may interact with diabetes drugs.

52. How does physical exercise affect blood glucose levels?

Physical exercise is an integral part of managing diabetes. It helps lower blood glucose levels by increasing insulin sensitivity and allowing cells to use glucose more efficiently. It also helps control weight, reduce stress and cardiovascular risk, improve overall well-being, and reduce the risk of complications. It is recommended to combine aerobic exercise with resistance training.

53. What role does fiber play in a person's diet with diabetes?

Fiber, especially soluble fiber, helps control blood sugar levels by slowing glucose absorption. Eating foods rich in fiber, such as whole grains, legumes, vegetables and fruits, improves digestive health, contributes to feelings of satiety, and aids in weight control.

54. What is hyperglycemia, and how is it managed?

Hyperglycemia is when blood glucose levels are too high. It is managed by adjusting medication, controlling diet, increasing physical activity, and regularly monitoring glucose levels.

55. What are the most common symptoms of hyperglycemia?

Symptoms may include excessive thirst, frequent urination, fatigue, blurred vision, and, if left untreated, can lead to serious complications.

56. What is non-ketotic hyperosmolar hyperglycemia?

It is an acute complication of type 2 diabetes characterized by extremely high blood glucose levels without the accumulation of ketones. Symptoms include extreme thirst, dehydration and confusion.

57. How does diabetes affect the kidneys?

Diabetes can damage the blood vessels in the kidneys, leading to a condition called diabetic nephropathy. This condition can progress to kidney failure if not controlled.

58. What is diabetic nephropathy, and how can it be prevented?

Diabetic nephropathy is a complication of diabetes that affects the kidneys. It is characterized by damage to the glomeruli, the kidney's filtration units, which can lead to kidney failure in advanced stages. Prevention includes strict glucose and blood pressure control and administering medications such as ACE inhibitors or angiotensin receptor blockers.

59. What is diabetic retinopathy?

Diabetic retinopathy is a complication of diabetes that affects the eyes. It is caused by damage to the retina's blood vessels caused by high blood glucose levels. If not treated properly, diabetic retinopathy can lead to vision problems and, in severe cases, blindness.

60. What are the symptoms of diabetic retinopathy?

Symptoms may include blurred vision, dark spots in the vision, and loss of vision.

61. How can diabetes affect the eyes in addition to diabetic retinopathy?

In addition to retinopathy, diabetes can increase the risk of cataracts, glaucoma and macular edema, which can affect vision in several ways.

62. How can artificial sweeteners affect people with diabetes?

Artificial sweeteners may offer a calorie-free alternative to sugar, but their impact on insulin and metabolism is debated, with some research concluding that they may affect the gut microbiota.

63. Does magnesium play a role in the management of diabetes?

Magnesium is essential for insulin function and glucose metabolism. Some research concludes that magnesium deficiency may increase the risk of developing type 2 diabetes.

64. What is the exchange diet for people with diabetes?

The exchange diet is a meal-planning method that helps people with diabetes control their carbohydrate, protein and fat intake. Foods are grouped into categories, and portions are exchanged within each group to maintain nutritional balance.

65. What is the relationship between diabetes and obesity?

Obesity is a significant risk factor for the development of type 2 diabetes. Excess body fat, especially around the abdomen, can increase insulin resistance, contributing to the development of the disease. Weight loss and a healthy weight help prevent and control type 2 diabetes.

66. What is insulin therapy in type 1 diabetes?

Insulin therapy is essential for people with type 1 diabetes because their bodies do not produce insulin. Exogenous insulin is administered through injections or an insulin pump to maintain blood glucose levels within the target range.

67. How is sleep related to diabetes management?

Adequate sleep is crucial for diabetes management. Lack of sleep or poor quality sleep affects blood glucose levels and increases insulin resistance. Establishing healthy sleep habits helps improve disease control.

68. What is fasting glucose, and why is it important?

Fasting glucose measures blood sugar levels after a fast of at least 8 hours. It is an essential test for diagnosing diabetes and assessing blood sugar control.

69. How does diabetes impact a person's daily life?

Diabetes requires ongoing management, including regular glucose monitoring, meal planning, physical activity, and medication. This can be challenging, but they can lead entire and active lives with proper education and support.

70. What is a continuous glucose meter (CGM)?

A continuous glucose meter is a device that monitors blood glucose levels constantly throughout the day in the body's interstitial fluid, providing real-time data. This helps people with diabetes adjust their treatment more precisely.

71. Is zinc essential for people with diabetes?

Zinc is involved in the synthesis, storage and release of insulin. A zinc deficiency can affect glucose control, and some studies conclude that supplementation may improve insulin function in people with diabetes.

72. How does diabetes affect cardiovascular health?

Diabetes increases the risk of cardiovascular diseases, such as coronary heart disease and stroke. This is due to factors such as hypertension, high cholesterol, and high blood glucose, which can damage the blood vessels and nerves that control the heart.

73. What is LADA type diabetes?

LADA (Latent Autoimmune Diabetes in Adults) is a form of autoimmune diabetes that develops in adults. It is often confused with type 2 diabetes but shares characteristics of type 1

74. What impact does chromium have on diabetes?

Chromium is a mineral that can improve insulin action and carbohydrate metabolism. Some studies conclude that chromium supplementation helps to improve glucose control in people with type 2 diabetes.

75. How important is education in diabetes management?

Diabetes education is crucial for helping people understand their condition, learn to manage their glucose levels, and make informed decisions about their health and treatment.

76. What is glucagon, and when is it used in diabetes?

Glucagon is a hormone that raises blood glucose levels. It is used in emergencies to treat severe hypoglycemia in people with diabetes, especially when they are unconscious or unable to consume carbohydrates.

77. What are incretins, and how do they help manage type 2 diabetes?

Incretins are hormones that help regulate blood glucose by stimulating insulin secretion and decreasing glucagon release. Drugs that mimic these hormones may improve glycemic control in type 2 diabetes.

78. What are the benefits of alpha-lipoic acid for people with diabetes?

Alpha-lipoic acid is an antioxidant that reduces oxidative stress and improves insulin sensitivity. It has also been studied for its potential to alleviate the symptoms of diabetic neuropathy.

79. How does genetics influence the risk of developing diabetes?

Genetics plays a role in the risk of developing type 1 and type 2 diabetes, with multiple genes involved in susceptibility and glucose metabolism. A family history of diabetes increases the risk, although environmental, dietary, and lifestyle factors are also crucial. Certain environmental factors are thought to trigger the autoimmune response that destroys pancreatic beta cells in type 1 diabetes.

80. What is MODY type diabetes?

MODY (Maturity Onset Diabetes of the Young) is a rare monogenic form of inherited diabetes usually diagnosed before the age of 25. It is characterized by defects in insulin secretion due to genetic mutations and is managed differently from type 1 or type 2 diabetes.

81. What are beta cells, and what is their function in

diabetes?

Beta cells are found in the islets of Langerhans of the pancreas and are responsible for producing insulin. In type 1 diabetes, the immune system destroys these cells, while in type 2 diabetes, they may not function properly.

82. What is a beta cell transplant, and how can it help people with type 1 diabetes?

A beta cell transplant involves transplanting insulin-producing cells into people with type 1 diabetes. This experimental technique seeks to restore the body's ability to produce insulin.

83. What is glucotoxicity, and how does it affect people with diabetes?

Glucotoxicity refers to the damage that high glucose levels can cause to the beta cells of the pancreas and other tissues. It can worsen insulin production and the progression of diabetes.

84. What recent innovations are there in the treatment of diabetes?

Recent innovations include insulin pumps with continuous glucose monitoring systems, artificial pancreas, mobile apps, and new oral and injectable medications that help monitor and manage glucose levels.

85. What is an insulin pump, and how does it work?

An insulin pump is a device that delivers insulin continuously through a small catheter inserted under the skin. It allows for more precise and flexible control of blood glucose levels.

86. What are continuous glucose sensors, and how do they work?

Continuous glucose monitors (CGM) constantly monitor glucose levels in interstitial fluid. They provide real-time data, which helps people with diabetes make informed decisions about their treatment.

87. What is a carbohydrate count, and how does it help people with diabetes?

Carbohydrate counting is a meal-planning technique that helps people with diabetes control their carbohydrate intake. By counting carbohydrate grams and adjusting insulin accordingly, better blood glucose control can be maintained.

88. What are the potential benefits of low-carbohydrate diets for people with diabetes?

Low-carbohydrate diets help control blood glucose levels, improve insulin sensitivity, and facilitate weight loss.

89. What are insulin analogs, and how do they differ from regular insulin?

Insulin analogs are modified forms of insulin designed to act faster or for a more extended period than regular insulin. They offer greater flexibility and control in managing glucose levels.

90. How can the Mediterranean diet benefit people with diabetes?

The Mediterranean diet, rich in fruits, vegetables, legumes, fish, and healthy fats, has been shown to improve blood glucose control and reduce the risk of cardiovascular complications in people with diabetes.

91. What is acanthosis nigricans, and its relation to diabetes?

Acanthosis nigricans is a skin condition characterized by dark, velvety areas, usually on the neck, armpits, and body folds. It is associated with insulin resistance and may be a sign of prediabetes or type 2 diabetes.

92. Can children develop diabetes?

Yes, children can develop diabetes. Type 1 diabetes is more common in children and adolescents, while type 2 diabetes is increasing among young people due to unhealthy diets and the rise in childhood obesity.

93. How is type 1 diabetes diagnosed in children?

Type 1 diabetes in children is diagnosed by blood tests that measure glucose levels. Symptoms may include excessive thirst, frequent urination, fatigue and unexplained weight loss.

94. What is a diabetes management plan, and what should it include?

A diabetes management plan is a personalized set of strategies to control the disease, including a meal plan, exercise regimen, glucose monitoring, and, if necessary, supplements, medication, or insulin.

95. What is continuous glucose monitoring, and what are its benefits?

Continuous glucose monitoring is a technology that provides frequent readings of blood glucose levels, helping people with diabetes maintain more accurate control and prevent episodes of hypoglycemia and hyperglycemia.

96. What role does the intestinal microbiota play in diabetes?

Gut microbiota can influence metabolism and inflammation, affecting the risk of developing insulin resistance and type 2 diabetes. Research in this field is ongoing to better understand these connections.

97. Are fruits safe for people with diabetes?

Fruits contain natural sugars but are rich in fiber, vitamins and minerals. They can be included in a person's diet with diabetes, but it is crucial to control portions and opt for fruits with a low glycemic index, such as berries and apples.

98. How can fenugreek help in the management of diabetes?

Fenugreek helps reduce blood glucose levels and improves glucose tolerance. Its seeds contain soluble fiber that slows digestion and carbohydrate absorption.

99. What is the importance of hydration in the management of diabetes?

Staying well hydrated is crucial for people with diabetes, as dehydration negatively affects blood sugar control. Drinking enough water helps maintain more stable glucose levels.

100. How can diabetes be managed during illness?

It is important to monitor glucose levels more frequently during an illness, adjust medication as needed, and stay well hydrated to effectively manage diabetes.

101. Is ginseng effective in controlling diabetes?

Ginseng has been studied for its ability to improve blood sugar regulation and increase insulin sensitivity. Although it shows potential, it should be used cautiously and under medical supervision.

102. How are diabetes and cholesterol related?

People with diabetes tend to have higher levels of LDL ("bad") cholesterol and triglycerides and lower levels of HDL ("good") cholesterol, which increases their risk of cardiovascular disease.

103. How does diabetes affect blood circulation?

Diabetes can damage blood vessels and nerves, which reduces blood circulation. This can lead to complications such as foot problems and peripheral arterial disease.

104. What are SGLT2 inhibitors, and how do they help treat diabetes?

SGLT2 inhibitors are a class of drugs that help lower blood glucose levels by increasing their excretion in the urine. They may also have additional cardiovascular and renal health benefits.

105. Is it safe to combine herbal treatments with diabetes medications?

It is not always safe to combine herbal treatments with diabetes medications, as some herbs may interact with the drugs and alter their effects. It is essential to consult a physician before combining treatments.

106. How can diabetes affect the autonomic nervous system?

Diabetes can damage the autonomic nervous system, which controls involuntary body functions such as blood pressure, digestion and heart rate, which can lead to complications such as gastroparesis and orthostatic hypotension.

107. What is diabetic gastroparesis, and how does it affect digestion?

Diabetic gastroparesis is a disorder in which the stomach empties slowly due to nerve damage, affecting digestion and blood glucose control.

108. What role does basal insulin play in the treatment of diabetes?

Basal insulin is a long-acting insulin that helps maintain stable blood glucose levels between meals and overnight in people with diabetes.

109. What role does vitamin D play in diabetes?

Vitamin D may influence insulin sensitivity and pancreatic beta cell function. Some studies conclude that adequate levels of vitamin D help improve glucose control.

110. Can cinnamon help reduce blood sugar levels?

Some scientific studies conclude that cinnamon can improve insulin sensitivity and reduce blood glucose levels. However, you must consult your doctor if you are under pharmacological treatment.

111. How can hormonal changes during puberty affect the management of diabetes in adolescents?

Hormonal changes during puberty can increase insulin resistance, which can make glucose control more difficult in adolescents with diabetes.

112. What is microalbuminuria, and what does it indicate in people with diabetes?

Microalbuminuria is the presence of small amounts of albumin in the urine. It can be an early sign of kidney damage in people with diabetes. Early detection and treatment are crucial to prevent the progression of kidney disease.

113. How does diabetes affect wound healing?

Diabetes can slow wound healing due to poor circulation, nerve damage and decreased immune function, which increases the risk of ulcers and other complications.

114. What is the effect of neem on diabetes?

Neem has been used in traditional medicine to control blood sugar. Scientific studies confirm hypoglycemic effects.

115. How can diabetes affect bone health?

Diabetes may increase the risk of osteoporosis and bone fractures due to altered calcium metabolism, chronic inflammation and microvascular damage.

116. What are GLP-1 analogs, and how do they help treat type 2 diabetes?

GLP-1 analogs mimic the action of the GLP-1 hormone, helping to improve insulin secretion, reduce blood glucose, and promote weight loss in people with type 2 diabetes.

117. Can diabetes affect hearing?

Yes, diabetes can increase the risk of hearing loss due to damage to the blood vessels and nerves of the inner ear.

118. What is insulin-related lipodystrophy?

Lipodystrophy is a condition that can occur in insulin users. It is characterized by changes in body fat distribution at sites of repeated insulin injection and can affect insulin absorption.

119. What are the effects of diabetes on the skin?

Diabetes can cause skin problems such as infections and itching, and conditions such as diabetic dermopathy and necrobiosis lipoidica.

120. What is diabetic dermopathy, and how does it manifest in the skin?

Diabetic dermopathy is a common skin condition in people with diabetes characterized by brown or reddish spots on the skin, usually on the legs. It is associated with changes in the small blood vessels.

121. How does diabetes affect cognitive function?

Diabetes, mainly if not well controlled, can increase the risk of cognitive impairment and dementia due to the effects of high glucose in the brain.

122. What is the Somogyi phenomenon?

The Somogyi phenomenon is a hyperglycemic rebound after a nocturnal hypoglycemia episode. It occurs when counter-regulatory hormones are released and raise blood glucose levels.

123. How can diabetes influence sexual health?

Diabetes can cause erectile dysfunction in men and arousal and lubrication problems in women due to nerve damage and poor blood circulation.

124. What is the glycemic load, and how does it relate to the diabetes diet?

Glycemic load is a measure that considers the quality and quantity of carbohydrates in food and their impact on blood glucose levels. It helps people with diabetes plan an appropriate diet.

125. How does diabetes affect nutrient absorption?

Diabetes can alter gastrointestinal motility and bowel function, affecting the absorption of certain nutrients, especially if there is autonomic neuropathy.

126. How can diabetes influence the risk of infections?

People with diabetes are at increased risk for infections due to impaired immune response, poor circulation, and high glucose levels that may favor bacterial growth.

127. How does diabetes affect heart health?

Diabetes can increase the risk of heart disease due to damage to blood vessels, increased cholesterol and high blood pressure.

128. Can diabetes influence the development of auto-immune diseases?

Type 1 diabetes, in particular, is associated with an increased risk of developing other autoimmune diseases, such as celiac disease and autoimmune thyroiditis.

129. Is omega-3 beneficial for people with diabetes?

Omega-3 fatty acids, found in oily fish and some supplements, can help reduce inflammation and improve cardiovascular health. This is especially important for people with diabetes, as they are at an increased risk of heart disease.

130. What is diabetes insipidus, and how is it different from diabetes mellitus?

Diabetes insipidus is characterized by the production of large amounts of dilute urine and excessive thirst. It is caused by problems in the production or action of the hormone vasopressin and is unrelated to glucose control.

131. What is body mass index (BMI) and its relationship to diabetes?

BMI is a measure of body fat based on weight and height. A high BMI, especially obesity, is closely related to an increased risk of developing type 2 diabetes.

132. What is the dawn phenomenon in diabetes?

The dawn phenomenon refers to a natural rise in blood glucose in the early morning due to hormonal changes. This rise may require adjustments in diabetes management.

133. What is autonomic neuropathy, and how does it manifest itself in diabetes?

Autonomic neuropathy affects the nerves that control involuntary body functions, such as digestion and blood pressure, and is a complication of diabetes that can cause digestive, cardiovascular, and other dysfunctions.

134. How is diabetes related to cancer risk?

Diabetes, especially type 2 diabetes, has been associated with an increased risk of certain types of cancer, possibly due to factors such as insulin resistance, chronic inflammation and elevated glucose levels.

SUGGESTED PRACTICAL PLAN

Managing diabetes, regardless of its type, requires a holistic approach that goes beyond simply controlling blood sugar levels. It means adopting healthy habits, caring for all aspects of your well-being, and prioritizing your overall quality of life. If you're navigating life with diabetes, I am here to support you every step of the way. Below is a complete guide filled with practical strategies to help you manage diabetes effectively and positively. Let's dive in!

‣ **Understand the Root Cause of Your Diabetes**: The first step in managing diabetes is understanding what's causing it and, when possible, addressing or minimizing the underlying triggering factors. This self-awareness is critical for taking preventive or corrective measures. For further insights, consult the chapter "Diabetes", particularly the sections "Causes" and "Symptoms Reduction and Prevention".

‣ **Nutrition: Your Greatest Ally**: Your diet plays a pivotal role in controlling diabetes. Some foods work to enhance your health, while others may hinder effective disease management. The chapters "Foods That Transform" and "Juices and Smoothies" provide detailed guidance and over 100 meal ideas tailored just for you. These resources will help you savor delicious, health-conscious meals, along with a variety of juices and shakes specially crafted to maintain balanced blood sugar levels.

‣ **Make Exercise a Non-Negotiable Habit**: Movement is essential–especially for managing diabetes! Regular physical activity not only helps you maintain a healthy weight but also improves your body's sensitivity to insulin. Strive for at least 150 minutes of moderate physical activity per week, such as walking, dancing, swimming, or cycling. Incorporating strength training exercises can amplify these benefits and further stabilize glucose levels. Remember, staying active doesn't have to feel like a chore–it can be both fun and incredibly rewarding!

▸ **Explore Supplements and Herbal Remedies**: Certain nutritional supplements may accelerate blood glucose regulation in your body. Additionally, herbal remedies can serve as a natural complement to your treatment plan, with specific medicinal plants offering supportive benefits. To learn more, explore the chapter "Medicinal Plants", where you'll discover valuable insights and guidance on complementary approaches.

▸ **Weight Management and Its Impact**: Maintaining a healthy weight is an essential cornerstone of diabetes management. Achieving this can significantly enhance your insulin sensitivity and support more stable blood sugar levels. Remember, consistent daily effort–no matter how small–can lead to substantial changes over time!

▸ **Keeping Stress in Check**: Stress is one of the most significant challenges to managing diabetes, as it has a direct impact on blood sugar levels. Incorporating stress management techniques such as meditation, mindfulness, deep breathing exercises, yoga, or tai chi can help promote both emotional and physical well-being. If you find yourself struggling with stress, don't hesitate to seek professional psychological support. Taking care of your mental health is a vital component of managing diabetes effectively.

▸ **The Power of Quality Sleep**: Getting enough restful sleep not only boosts your energy levels but also plays a crucial role in blood sugar regulation. Poor sleep or sleep deprivation can disrupt your glucose levels. To avoid this, establish a consistent sleep routine, optimize your sleep environment, and prioritize adequate rest.

▸ **Consult About Your Medications**: If you're taking medications for diabetes or any other medical condition, and you notice new or worsening symptoms, consult your doctor promptly. It might be necessary to adjust your dosage or modify your treatment plan to better suit your needs. Always follow professional medical advice, and never make changes to your medication regimen without consulting your healthcare provider.

▸ **Regular Glucose Monitoring**: Monitoring your blood sugar regularly is an invaluable practice to better understand how your body reacts to various factors such as food, exercise, supplements, or medicinal plants. Work with your doctor to determine the optimal frequency for monitoring. Keeping a detailed journal of your results can help you make better-informed decisions about your diabetes management.

Managing Other Health Concerns

If you're facing other health conditions alongside diabetes—such as insomnia, anxiety, arthritis, hypertension, or gastritis—you may find additional support in resources tailored to those specific concerns. Practical recommendations on food, supplements, and medicinal plants are available in the following titles, which may help improve your overall well-being:

▸ **Acid reflux**. Foods, Supplements and Herbs
▸ **Anxiety**. Foods, Supplements and Herbs
▸ **Arthritis**. Foods, Supplements and Herbs
▸ **Cholesterol**. Foods, Supplements and Herbs
▸ **Fibromyalgia**. Foods, Supplements and Herbs
▸ **Gastritis**. Foods, Supplements and Herbs
▸ **Hypertension**. Foods, Supplements and Herbs
▸ **Insomnia**. Foods, Supplements and Herbs
▸ **Osteoarthritis**. Foods, Supplements and Herbs
▸ **Varicose veins**. Foods, Supplements and Herbs

Remember, managing diabetes is a continuous process that involves learning, adapting, and making informed choices. Every step, no matter how small, is progress toward a healthier, more balanced, and fulfilling life. You've got this!

NUTRITIONAL SUPPLEMENTS

"Supplements are little allies that give us an extra boost on our path to optimal health" (Dr. Mark Hyman)

Nutritional supplements have become a valuable ally in the pursuit of better health and an enhanced quality of life. These options–available in various user-friendly formats such as tablets, capsules, powders, or easily consumable liquids–are purposefully designed to complement your daily nutrition by delivering essential nutrients that can be challenging to obtain through regular meals alone. Packed with powerful components like vitamins, minerals, amino acids, antioxidants, and other bioactive compounds, these supplements are expertly formulated in precise proportions to meet the unique needs of every individual–even when the demands are high. Whether you're navigating restrictive diets, facing nutritional gaps, or coping with increased physical or mental demands, supplements can provide the extra support your body needs.

Beyond simply filling in nutritional gaps, supplements offer an array of tailored benefits to suit diverse lifestyles and health challenges. They can help boost energy, improve physical performance, support those managing fast-paced lives, and provide practical solutions for staying balanced and resilient. Their significance often becomes even more apparent during times of illness, specific health conditions, or chronic issues. In these situations, supplements do more than complement a diet–they can actively help restore altered functions, ease symptoms, and assist in more complex recovery processes. They serve as companions in the pursuit of health, helping you sustain and rebuild your vitality.

Effectively integrating supplements into your routine requires thoughtful use grounded in science and, when needed, professional guidance. By understanding their benefits and approaching them with care, supplements can evolve into powerful tools for improving your overall well-being in a sustainable and meaningful way. Remember–every step you take toward caring for your body is a step closer to feeling stronger, more energized, and more capable of facing life's challenges with confidence. Take that step today. Your path to better health begins with small but impactful choices!

Essential Precautions

Understanding the risks associated with supplements is vital, as they can sometimes cause side effects, have contraindications, or interact with medications. It's important to thoroughly review the potential adverse effects detailed at the end of this chapter. Take a moment to assess your overall health and avoid any supplements that could conflict with the medications you're currently taking or exacerbate existing medical conditions. Prioritizing this step ensures a safer and more effective approach to improving your well-being.

Essential Information on the Use of Supplements

Diabetes is a condition that requires diligent and comprehensive management to maintain blood sugar levels within healthy ranges. While certain supplements and natural products can support the well-being of individuals with diabetes, their use should always be approached with caution and responsibility.

Here, we will outline the essential considerations to take into account before incorporating supplements into your diabetes management plan:

▸ **Please consult with your physician**: Before incorporating any supplement into your treatment regimen, it is essential to consult with a physician. They can evaluate the benefits and risks, considering your health and current drug treatment.

▸ **Constant glucose monitoring**: The supplements discussed below affect blood glucose levels. It is essential to regularly monitor your glucose levels to detect any changes and respond appropriately.

‣ **Medication adjustment by your medical specialist**: The following supplements have a hypoglycemic effect and often potentiate the action of antidiabetic drugs, which may require a dosage adjustment. Your physician may need to modify your treatment or adjust doses to avoid episodes of hypoglycemia.

‣ **Side effects and adverse reactions**: Some supplements may cause side effects in some people or interact with medications. Discard those you should not use due to health conditions or medical treatments.

Nutritional Supplements and Diabetes

Effectively managing diabetes requires a well-rounded approach that combines a nutritious diet, regular physical activity, and strict adherence to prescribed medical treatments. In addition to these foundational strategies, many people explore the use of nutritional supplements as a valuable support in their comprehensive diabetes management plan. These supplements have the potential to enhance insulin sensitivity, stabilize blood sugar levels, and contribute to overall metabolic health.

That said, while supplements can be a helpful addition, it is crucial to use them responsibly. Their effectiveness and safety can vary from person to person, and they should always be taken under the guidance of a qualified healthcare professional.

In this section, we will delve into some of the most notable and commonly used supplements for managing diabetes. These supplements are listed alphabetically and include thorough details regarding their potential benefits, recommended dosages, optimal usage guidelines, estimated timeframes to see results, and the recommended duration for safe use. The supplements discussed include **alpha-lipoic acid, berberine, cinnamon, chromium, fenugreek, gymnema, ginseng, magnesium, omega-3 fatty acids, vitamin D, and zinc**.

By exploring this section, you'll gain valuable insights that can help you use these supplements in a safe and effective manner. Incorporating them thoughtfully into your routine can support a holistic and personalized approach to diabetes management. Let's dive into the details to discover how these supplements can positively impact your well-being!

Alpha-lipoic acid

Alpha lipoic acid (ALA) is a potent antioxidant found naturally in the body and obtained through food and supplements. It is known for improving insulin sensitivity and reducing oxidative stress, making it particularly interesting to people with diabetes. Below are the benefits and considerations for using ALA.

Diabetes benefits

‣ Improved insulin sensitivity: ALA helps cells use glucose more efficiently, improving insulin sensitivity and helping to control blood sugar levels.

‣ Reduction of oxidative stress: As a potent antioxidant, ALA combats free radical damage, which is more prevalent in people with diabetes and contributes to developing complications.

‣ Diabetic neuropathy relief: ALA has been studied for its ability to relieve symptoms of diabetic neuropathy, a common complication of diabetes that causes pain and numbness in the extremities.

‣ Cardiovascular protection: By reducing oxidative stress and improving endothelial function, ALA helps protect against cardiovascular disease, which is at an elevated risk in people with diabetes.

Recommended dosage

The dosage of alpha lipoic acid may vary according to the purpose of treatment. Scientific studies typically use 300 mg to 600 mg per day for diabetes and diabetic neuropathy. However, it is essential not to exceed the recommended dose without the supervision of a healthcare professional, as higher doses do not always equate to better results and may increase the risk of side effects.

Posology

The administration of alpha lipoic acid can be flexible, but there are some general recommendations:

Frequency: To maintain stable levels in the body, the daily dose can be divided into two or three doses.

Timing: It can be taken in the morning or the afternoon. Some people prefer to take it in the evening, mainly if it is used for neuropathy.

Although ALA is best absorbed on an empty stomach, some people take it with food to minimize gastrointestinal discomfort.

Average action onset time
Although the onset of action may vary from person to person, many people notice its antioxidant effects and improvements in insulin sensitivity and neuropathy symptoms within a few weeks of regular use. Therefore, consistency with supplementation is essential to evaluating its efficacy.

Maximum time of continuous use
There is no strict consensus on the maximum time alpha lipoic acid can be used, but it is generally considered safe for long-term use under physician supervision. However, periodic evaluations are advisable to determine its continued effectiveness and safety, especially if used in conjunction with other diabetes treatments.

Berberine

Berberine is a bioactive compound in several plants, including barberry, goldenseal and coptis. Traditional Chinese and Ayurvedic medicine have used it for its therapeutic properties. Recently, it has gained attention for its benefits in managing diabetes, as it can regulate glucose metabolism and improve insulin sensitivity.

Diabetes benefits
‣ Blood glucose regulation: Reduces blood glucose levels by improving insulin sensitivity and decreasing glucose production in the liver.

‣ Improved lipid profile: Besides its effect on glucose, it helps reduce LDL cholesterol and triglyceride levels, which benefits cardiovascular health in people with diabetes.

‣ Increased insulin sensitivity: Insulin acts on AMP-activated protein kinase (AMPK), an enzyme crucial for energy metabolism, thus improving cell glucose uptake.

‣ Anti-inflammatory and antioxidant properties: It also possesses properties that reduce oxidative stress and inflammation, conditions that are commonly associated with diabetes.

Recommended dosage

The dose of berberine used for managing diabetes generally ranges from 900 mg to 1,500 mg per day, divided into several doses. The maximum recommended dose can be as high as 2,000 mg per day, but this should be done under the supervision of a healthcare professional to minimize the risk of side effects.

Posology

Berberine should be taken in several doses throughout the day to maximize its absorption and efficacy:

Frequency: It is common to divide the daily dose into two or three doses, for example, 500 mg three times a day.

Timing: It is recommended to be taken with meals to improve absorption and reduce the risk of adverse gastrointestinal effects. Taking it before meals helps to control postprandial glucose spikes (the blood glucose level measured after eating).

Average action onset time

Many studies and reports conclude that effects on blood glucose usually begin to be seen within a few weeks of regular use. However, it is essential to remember that the response may be individual and that consistency in administration is key to assessing effectiveness.

Maximum time of continuous use

Berberine is generally safe for long-term use when taken at recommended doses. However, due to the lack of extensive long-term studies, people using it to manage diabetes should do so under the supervision of a healthcare professional.

Cinnamon

Cinnamon is a spice known for its culinary and medicinal properties. Recently, it has gained attention for its potential to help manage diabetes.

Diabetes benefits
‣ Reduction of blood glucose levels: Several scientific studies conclude that it helps reduce fasting blood glucose levels. This is due to its ability to improve insulin sensitivity, allowing cells to utilize glucose better.

‣ Improved insulin sensitivity: It acts as an insulin modulator, enhancing its effectiveness and helping cells to absorb glucose more efficiently.

‣ Antioxidant properties: It contains antioxidant compounds that reduce oxidative stress, a condition frequently associated with diabetes.

‣ Anti-inflammatory effects: Chronic inflammation is a common factor in type 2 diabetes, and cinnamon's anti-inflammatory properties help reduce it.

‣ Improved lipid profile: Some studies have shown that it helps reduce LDL cholesterol and triglyceride levels, which benefits diabetics' cardiovascular health.

Recommended dosage
The dose of cinnamon used in studies varies, but generally, a dose of 1 to 6 grams per day is recommended. It is essential to avoid excessive consumption, as high doses can be toxic due to coumarin, especially in Cassia cinnamon. Ceylon cinnamon has lower levels of coumarin and may be a safer option.

Posology

Frequency: Dividing the daily dose into two or three intakes is recommended.

Timing: Taking it with meals is beneficial for controlling postprandial glucose spikes (the blood glucose level measured after eating). It can be added to food and beverages or taken as a supplement.

Dosage form: It can be consumed as a powder or capsule supplement.

Average action onset time

The time of onset of action may vary among individuals. Some studies indicate that effects on blood glucose usually begin to be observed after several weeks of regular use. The response may depend on factors such as diet, physical activity level, and severity of insulin resistance.

Maximum time of continuous use

Cinnamon is generally safe for long-term use when consumed at recommended doses. However, due to the lack of long-term studies, it is recommended that people using cinnamon for diabetes management do so under the supervision of a healthcare professional.

Chromium

Chromium is an essential mineral in metabolizing carbohydrates, fats, and proteins. Its most studied form in the context of diabetes is chromium picolinate. It has been investigated for its potential to improve insulin sensitivity and aid in blood glucose control.

Diabetes benefits

▸ Improved insulin sensitivity: Chromium is known to enhance insulin's action, which helps improve glucose uptake by cells and reduce blood glucose levels.

▸ Blood glucose control: Some scientific studies have shown that chromium supplementation helps reduce fasting blood glucose levels and improves overall glycemic control in people with diabetes.

‣ Metabolism regulation: It plays a role in the metabolism of macronutrients, helping regulate blood sugar levels and contributing to weight control, which is crucial for managing diabetes.

‣ Cholesterol reduction: Some studies conclude that it positively affects cholesterol levels, which benefits cardio-vascular health in people with diabetes.

Recommended dosage

Dosage may vary depending on the preparation and concentration of the supplement. However, doses commonly studied in diabetes research range from 200 to 1000 micrograms (mcg) per day of chromium picolinate. It is essential to stay within the recommended dose.

Posology

Frequency: Generally taken once or twice a day.

Timing: May be taken with meals to improve absorption and minimize the risk of stomach upset.

Dosage form: It is available in capsules, tablets, or as part of multivitamins.

Average action onset time

The time of onset of action in improving insulin sensitivity and glucose control may vary. Some people may notice changes in blood glucose after several weeks to months of regular use. Response to chromium may depend on individual factors, including diet, level of physical activity, and degree of insulin resistance.

Maximum time of continuous use

Chromium is generally considered safe for long-term use when taken at recommended doses. However, due to variability in individual response and the lack of very long-term studies, it is advised that individuals taking chromium supplements do so under the supervision of a healthcare professional.

Fenugreek

Fenugreek has been a medicinal plant used for centuries in various cultures to treat different health conditions, including diabetes. Its seeds are rich in soluble fiber, bioactive compounds and galactomannans, which help improve blood glucose control and insulin resistance.

Diabetes benefits
‣ Improved blood glucose control: Its high soluble fiber content helps reduce blood glucose levels, especially after meals, by slowing down the absorption of carbohydrates in the intestine.

‣ Increased insulin sensitivity: Some scientific studies conclude that it improves insulin sensitivity, which is beneficial for people with diabetes who have insulin resistance.

‣ Reduction of cholesterol and triglycerides: In addition to its effects on glucose, it helps to improve the lipid profile, reducing LDL cholesterol and triglycerides, which is beneficial for cardiovascular health.

‣ Antioxidant and anti-inflammatory properties: The antioxidant compounds help reduce oxidative stress and inflammation, which are often associated with diabetes.

Recommended dosage
Dosage may vary depending on the preparation and the purpose of the treatment. However, commonly recommended doses for managing diabetes range from 5 to 25 grams of seeds daily or 500 to 1,000 milligrams of fenugreek extract daily. Do not exceed these doses to avoid possible side effects.

Posology
Frequency: It can be taken once or several times a day.

Timing: It is recommended to be taken with meals to maximize its benefits on postprandial glucose control (the blood glucose level measured after a meal).

Dosage form: Fenugreek is available in whole seeds, powder, capsules, or liquid extract. The seeds can be soaked in water and consumed directly or mixed in food.

Average action onset time

The time of fenugreek's onset of action may vary among people. Some studies conclude that effects on blood glucose may begin to be observed after several weeks of regular use. The response may depend on diet, physical activity level and insulin resistance.

Maximum time of continuous use

Fenugreek is generally safe for long-term use when consumed at recommended doses. However, due to the lack of very long-term studies, it is recommended that people using it for diabetes management do so under the supervision of a healthcare professional.

Ginseng

Ginseng is a plant that has been used in traditional Asian medicine for thousands of years. There are several species of ginseng, with Asian ginseng (Panax ginseng) and American ginseng (Panax quinquefolius) being the most studied regarding diabetes. Ginseng contains ginsenosides, a bioactive compound responsible for its health benefits, including diabetes management.

Diabetes benefits

‣ Improved insulin sensitivity: This helps improve insulin sensitivity, which allows the cells to utilize glucose more efficiently and reduces blood sugar levels.

‣ Reduction of blood glucose levels: Some scientific studies have shown that ginseng helps lower fasting blood glucose levels and improve overall glycemic control in people with diabetes.

‣ Anti-inflammatory and antioxidant properties: Ginsenosides possess anti-inflammatory and antioxidant properties, which help reduce oxidative stress and inflammation, factors that often complicate diabetes.

‣ Improved lipid profile: It also improves the lipid profile, reducing LDL cholesterol and triglyceride levels, which benefits cardiovascular health in people with diabetes.

Recommended dosage

The dosage of a supplement may vary depending on its form and concentration. However, the recommended dose for diabetes management generally ranges from 200 to 400 milligrams of standardized extract per day. Adherence to these recommended dosages is essential.

Posology

Frequency: Ginseng is usually taken once or twice a day.

Timing: It can be taken in the morning and/or at noon to avoid possible insomnia problems, as it may have a stimulating effect.

Dosage form: It is available in capsules, tablets, liquid extracts, or dried roots to prepare infusions.

Average action onset time

Improvements in blood glucose levels and insulin sensitivity usually begin to be noticed after weeks to months of regular use. The response may depend on diet, physical activity level and insulin resistance.

Maximum time of continuous use

Ginseng is generally considered safe for medium-term use, but due to the lack of very long-term studies, it is recommended to use it for up to three months, followed by a break of one to two weeks. This helps prevent possible side effects and maintains the supplement's effectiveness. It is essential to use ginseng under the supervision of a health professional.

Gymnema

Gymnema (Gymnema sylvestre) is a plant native to India that has been used in traditional medicine for centuries, especially in diabetes management. Its leaves contain bioactive compounds, such as gymnemic acid, which have been shown to help regulate blood sugar levels and improve insulin sensitivity.

Diabetes benefits

‣ Reduction of blood sugar levels: Gymnema helps to lower blood glucose levels, especially after meals, by interfering with the absorption of sugar in the intestine.

‣ Improved insulin sensitivity: Contributes to improving the sensitivity of cells to insulin, thus facilitating glucose utilization in the body and helping maintain blood sugar levels within a healthy range.

‣ Decreased sugar cravings: Gymnema reduces cravings for sweet foods, which is particularly beneficial for people with diabetes who struggle with sugar cravings.

‣ Antioxidant properties: Its compounds also possess antioxidant properties, which help reduce oxidative stress, which can complicate diabetes and contribute to the onset of complications.

Recommended dosage

The dosage may vary depending on the supplement's form and concentration. Generally, a daily dose of 200 to 400 milligrams of standardized Gymnema extract containing at least 25% gymnemic acid is recommended.

Posology

Frequency: Gymnema is usually taken once or twice a day.

Timing: To maximize absorption, it is recommended that you take the first dose on an empty stomach in the morning and a second dose before lunch or dinner.

Dosage form: It is available in capsules, tablets, liquid extracts, or powder for infusions.

Average action onset time

The effects on blood glucose levels and insulin sensitivity may begin to be noticeable 1 to 2 weeks after starting treatment. However, continued use and regular glucose level monitoring are recommended for optimal results.

Maximum time of continuous use
It is recommended to use Gymnema continuously for up to three months, followed by a break of at least one month. This rest period is essential for the body to adapt and avoid desensitization to its effects.

Magnesium

Magnesium is essential in numerous physiological processes, including regulating glucose metabolism and insulin function. Research concludes that there is a significant relationship between magnesium levels and the risk of developing type 2 diabetes. Magnesium deficiency is common in people with diabetes and can exacerbate glycemic control and complicate disease management.

Diabetes benefits
‣ Improved insulin sensitivity: Magnesium is crucial for insulin action, and its supplementation often enhances insulin sensitivity, facilitating better regulation of blood glucose levels.

‣ Blood glucose control: Magnesium supplementation has been shown to help reduce fasting blood glucose levels and improve overall glycemic control in people with diabetes.

‣ Reduced risk of cardiovascular complications: It helps regulate blood pressure and improves lipid profiles, reducing the risk of cardiovascular complications, which are common in people with diabetes.

‣ Anti-inflammatory properties: Its anti-inflammatory properties help reduce chronic inflammation associated with insulin resistance and diabetes.

The different magnesium compounds: the most and the least laxative.
Magnesium is an essential mineral that provides many benefits and plays numerous roles in body health. It reduces pain, muscle and nerve function, improves sleep, regulates blood

pressure, and supports the immune system. However, some magnesium compounds have laxative effects, which can be a problem for people prone to diarrhea.

Among the different types of magnesium supplements, magnesium citrate, magnesium chloride, and magnesium hydroxide (commonly found in antacids such as milk of magnesia) tend to have more pronounced laxative effects. These types of magnesium attract water to the intestine, which increases intestinal motility and may cause diarrhea in some people. Take any of these compounds if you suffer from constipation, as they will help make your stools less dry and hard. The most laxative compound of the three is usually magnesium chloride.

In contrast, magnesium glycinate is a magnesium compound considered less laxative. Therefore, it may be more suitable for people with diarrhea problems.

Magnesium glycinate combines magnesium with glycine, an amino acid. It is one of the best-tolerated forms of magnesium regarding gastrointestinal effects. Glycine is a stabilizing agent that can help minimize laxative effects and improve magnesium absorption.

People with diarrhea problems or gastrointestinal sensitivity should start with low doses of magnesium and gradually increase according to their tolerance.

Recommended dosage
The dosage may vary depending on the form of the supplement and individual needs. Generally, the recommended daily dose for adults with diabetes is 300 to 400 milligrams.

Posology
Frequency: Magnesium can be taken once or twice a day.

Timing: It can be taken at any time of the day, but some people prefer to take it in the evening due to its relaxing effect, which can help improve sleep quality.

Dosage form: It is available in various forms, including magnesium oxide, citrate, chloride, and glycinate. Magnesium citrate is one of the most bioavailable forms and is commonly recommended.

Average action onset time

The time to the onset of action may vary depending on the individual and the level of deficiency present. Insulin sensitivity and blood glucose control improvements usually begin to be seen after several weeks of continuous supplementation. However, some benefits, such as improved sleep quality or reduced muscle cramping, are usually noticed more quickly.

Maximum time of continuous use

Magnesium is generally safe for long-term use when consumed at recommended doses.

Omega-3

Omega-3 fatty acids are essential polyunsaturated fats for maintaining cardiovascular and metabolic health. The primary dietary forms of omega-3s are eicosapentaenoic acid (EPA) and docosahexaenoic acid (DHA), which are found primarily in fatty fish, and alpha-linolenic acid (ALA), which is found in plant sources. Omega-3 supplements, usually in fish oil, have been studied for their potential benefits for people with diabetes.

Diabetes benefits

‣ Improved cardiovascular health: People with diabetes have an increased risk of cardiovascular disease. Omega-3s help reduce triglyceride levels, lower blood pressure, improve endothelial function, and reduce cardiovascular risk.

‣ Reduction of inflammation: Chronic inflammation is an underlying factor in insulin resistance and the development of type 2 diabetes. Omega-3s have anti-inflammatory properties that help moderate this inflammation.

‣ Improved insulin sensitivity: Some studies conclude it enhances insulin sensitivity.

‣ Retinal health benefits: People with diabetes are at risk of developing eye complications, such as diabetic retinopathy. Omega-3s, which have anti-inflammatory and cell membrane-protective properties, help protect eye health.

Recommended dosage

Dosage may vary depending on individual needs and health goals. For heart and metabolic health, dosages typically range from 500 to 3,000 milligrams of EPA and DHA daily. It is essential not to exceed 3,000 milligrams without the supervision of a healthcare professional, as high doses may increase the risk of bleeding.

Posology

Frequency: They are usually taken once or twice a day.

Timing: It is recommended to take it with meals to improve absorption and minimize possible side effects, such as reflux or a fishy taste.

Dosage form: Omega-3s are available in fish oil capsules, krill oil, and liquid forms. Capsules are the most common and easiest to consume.

Average action onset time

It varies depending on the individual and the specific effect being observed. Cardiovascular benefits, such as triglyceride reduction, usually begin to be seen after several weeks to months of consistent use. Effects on inflammation may also require a similar time to be noticeable.

Maximum time of continuous use

Supplements are generally safe for long-term use when consumed at recommended doses. However, it is essential to monitor total fat intake and consult a healthcare professional, especially if taking anticoagulant medication, as omega-3s may affect blood clotting.

Vitamin D

Vitamin D is a fat-soluble vitamin crucial for calcium regulation and maintaining bone health. Its impact on the immune system, inflammation and glucose metabolism has also been investigated, making it a nutrient of interest in diabetes. Vitamin D deficiency is common in many populations and has been associated with an increased risk of developing type 2 diabetes.

Diabetes benefits

‣ Improved insulin sensitivity: Vitamin D can influence the function of the pancreas's beta cells, which are responsible for insulin production. Studies have concluded that it can improve insulin sensitivity and thus help control blood glucose levels.

‣ Reduced risk of type 2 diabetes: Some scientific studies have found that adequate vitamin D levels may be associated with a lower risk of developing type 2 diabetes.

‣ Anti-inflammatory properties: Its anti-inflammatory properties reduce chronic inflammation, which contributes to insulin resistance and the progression of diabetes.

‣ Improves bone and overall health: It is essential for calcium absorption and maintaining bone health, especially in people with diabetes who may be at increased risk for bone complications.

Recommended dosage

The recommended dose may vary according to age, health status, and serum levels. Generally, 600 to 800 IU (International Units) per day are recommended for adults. However, some people may need higher doses to correct a deficiency under the supervision of a health professional. The maximum tolerable dose is generally set at 4,000 IU per day for adults. Due to the risk of toxicity, it is essential not to exceed this dose without medical supervision.

Posology

Frequency: Generally taken once a day.

Timing: It is recommended to take it with a fat-containing meal. This is because it is a fat-soluble vitamin whose absorption improves in the presence of fat.

Dosage form: It is available in various forms, including capsules, tablets, liquids, and in combination with calcium.

Average action onset time
The time required to observe the effects may vary. Correcting a vitamin D deficiency and improving insulin sensitivity may take several weeks to months, depending on the initial levels and dose administered. Changes in bone health and glucose control may require long-term monitoring.

Maximum time of continuous use
Vitamin D can be taken safely in the long term at recommended doses. However, regular testing of vitamin D blood levels is advisable to ensure optimal levels and avoid toxicity, especially if high doses are being used. Long-term supplementation should be under the supervision of your doctor.

Zinc

Zinc is an essential mineral for several biological functions, including carbohydrate metabolism and insulin regulation. In the context of diabetes, zinc supplementation may offer several benefits:

Diabetes benefits
▸ Improved insulin sensitivity: Helps improve insulin sensitivity, which means the body uses insulin more efficiently to lower blood glucose levels.

▸ Regulation of glucose metabolism: It has been shown to influence insulin production, storage and release, facilitating better glucose level control.

▸ Antioxidant properties: Oxidative stress contributes to diabetes complications. Zinc has antioxidant properties that help reduce cell damage.

▸ Wound healing: People with diabetes may experience problems with wound healing. Zinc is crucial for tissue repair and improves healing.

Recommended dosage

The recommended daily dose varies according to age, sex, and individual conditions. For adults, 8-11 mg is generally recommended. However, for therapeutic purposes, some people may take up to 40 mg per day, which is the tolerable upper limit established by health authorities. To avoid adverse effects, it is essential not to exceed this amount.

Posology

Zinc can be taken at any time of the day, but to maintain stable levels in the body, it is best to be consistent with the time of intake. It is best absorbed on an empty stomach, but some people may experience stomach upset. If discomfort is experienced, it is recommended to take it with meals.

Average action onset time

Generally, glucose levels and insulin sensitivity improvements can be observed after several weeks of continued use. However, antioxidant effects and wound-healing benefits may take longer to manifest.

Maximum time of continuous use

There is no specific limit for the continued use of zinc supplements as long as the maximum recommended dose of 40 mg daily is not exceeded. However, periodic evaluations with a health professional are advised to ensure that no side effects or drug interactions occur.

Adverse Effects, Contraindications, and Interactions

Before adding the recommended supplements to your routine, it is crucial to understand the potential adverse effects that may affect your health. Take the time to thoroughly review this section to ensure their safe and responsible use.

Alpha lip oic acid

▸ **Side effects:**

Some side effects may include nausea, skin rashes, or dizziness.

In people with diabetes, alpha lipoic acid can cause a decrease in blood glucose levels, which is beneficial, but can also increase the risk of hypoglycemia if sugar levels are not adequately monitored.

‣ Contraindications:

Its use is not recommended in people who are deficient in thiamine (vitamin B1), such as those with chronic alcohol abuse, as it may worsen the deficiency.

‣ Interactions:

It may interact with diabetes medications, increasing the risk of hypoglycemia. People with diabetes must monitor their blood sugar levels if they are taking alpha lipoic acid along with drugs such as insulin or sulfonylureas.

It may also interact with thyroid medications, so caution should be exercised and a healthcare professional consulted.

Berberine

‣ Side effects:

Side effects may include gastrointestinal problems such as diarrhea, constipation, gas and stomach pain.

For people with diabetes, berberine can help lower blood sugar levels, but there is a risk of hypoglycemia if glucose levels are not adequately monitored, especially if taken with other diabetes medications.

‣ Contraindications:

Due to the lack of data on its safety, it is not recommended for pregnant or lactating women.

‣ Interactions:

It may interact with diabetes medications, potentiating their effects and increasing the risk of hypoglycemia. It is crucial for people with diabetes to regularly monitor their blood glucose if they are using berberine together with medications.

It may also interact with certain antibiotics and other metabolized drugs in the liver, so use caution and consult your doctor or pharmacist.

Chromium

▶ Side effects:

In general, chromium picolinate is considered safe when taken in appropriate doses. However, side effects may include stomach upset, allergic reactions, dizziness, or headaches.

Chromium picolinate may help improve insulin sensitivity and lower blood glucose levels in people with diabetes. However, it is crucial to be aware of the potential risk of hypoglycemia, especially if taking medications to lower blood sugar.

▶ Contraindications:

People with kidney or liver problems should be cautious when using it, as it could aggravate these conditions.

▶ Interactions:

It may interact with diabetes medications, such as insulin or sulfonylureas, increasing the risk of hypoglycemia. People with diabetes must monitor their blood glucose levels if they are using this supplement.

It may also interact with medications that affect the thyroid, so caution and consultation with a physician or pharmacist are recommended.

Cinnamon

▶ Side effects:

Most people can safely consume cinnamon in standard dietary amounts. However, a compound called coumarin in Cassia cinnamon can irritate the mouth and lips and risk liver damage in high or concentrated doses.

For people with diabetes, there is a possibility that consumption of cinnamon may help lower blood sugar levels, which is beneficial, but may increase the risk of hypoglycemia if combined with diabetes medications.

▶ Contraindications:

People with liver disease should be cautious when consuming Cassia cinnamon due to its coumarin content, which can be harmful to the liver.

▶ Interactions:

It can potentiate the effects of diabetes medications, which could lead to dangerously low blood sugar levels. Therefore, people with diabetes must monitor their glucose levels if they use cinnamon and their medications.

It may also interact with other supplements and medications that affect the liver, so caution and medical or pharmaceutical consultation is recommended.

Fenugreek

▸ Side effects:

It is generally safe when consumed in dietary amounts, but in higher doses or as a supplement, it can cause side effects such as gastrointestinal discomfort, diarrhea, bloating and gas.

For people with diabetes, fenugreek may help lower blood glucose levels. However, this means that there is a potential risk of hypoglycemia, especially if taken with diabetes medications.

▸ Contraindications:

Its use is not recommended in pregnant women, as it may induce uterine contractions.

People with allergies to peanuts or chickpeas should be cautious, as fenugreek belongs to the same family of plants.

▸ Interactions:

Fenugreek may potentiate the effects of diabetes medications, which can lead to low blood sugar levels. Therefore, people with diabetes must monitor their glucose levels if they are using fenugreek in addition to their medications.

It may also interact with anticoagulants and drugs that affect blood clotting, so caution is advised.

Ginseng

▸ Side effects:

Ginseng is generally safe for most people when consumed in moderate doses. However, some may experience side effects such as insomnia, nervousness, headaches, stomach upset, and changes in blood pressure.

Ginseng may help lower blood glucose levels in people with diabetes. While this can be beneficial, it also increases the risk of hypoglycemia, especially if taken along with diabetes medications.

‣ Contraindications:

Its use is not recommended in pregnant or lactating women due to the lack of conclusive studies on its safety in these stages.

People with autoimmune diseases or taking immunosuppressants should be cautious, as ginseng may stimulate the immune system.

‣ Interactions:

It can interact with diabetes medications, increasing the risk of low blood sugar levels. Therefore, people with diabetes must monitor their glucose levels if they are using ginseng along with their medications.

It may also interact with anticoagulants, blood pressure medications, and medications that affect the central nervous system, so caution and medical or pharmaceutical consultations are recommended.

Gymnema

‣ Side effects:

Gymnema is generally well tolerated, but some people may experience stomach upset, nausea, diarrhea and skin rashes. These effects tend to be mild and temporary.

For people with diabetes, it helps lower blood glucose levels, but this carries a potential risk of hypoglycemia, especially if combined with anti-diabetic drugs.

‣ Contraindications:

It is not recommended during pregnancy and lactation because there are no studies on its safety in these conditions.

Also, people with a history of eating disorders should exercise caution when using it.

‣ Interactions:

Gymnema can potentiate the effects of anti-diabetic medications, resulting in low blood sugar levels. Therefore, people with diabetes must monitor their glucose levels regularly if they use cinema along with their medications.

In addition, it may interact with other herbal supplements that affect glucose and medications that modulate blood pressure, so caution is advised when combining treatments.

Magnesium

▸ **Side effects:**

Magnesium is generally safe for most people when consumed in adequate amounts. However, in high doses, it can cause side effects such as diarrhea, nausea, and abdominal cramps.

For people with diabetes, magnesium may improve insulin sensitivity and blood sugar control. However, the recommended dose should not be exceeded to avoid adverse effects.

▸ **Contraindications:**

People with kidney disease should exercise caution when taking magnesium supplements, as their ability to eliminate excess magnesium may be compromised.

▸ **Interactions:**

It can interact with certain medications, such as antibiotics and osteoporosis medications, reducing their effectiveness. Therefore, it is essential to take them at different times of the day.

There are no known direct interactions with diabetes medications, but monitoring blood glucose levels when introducing a new supplement is always advisable.

Omega-3

▸ **Side effects:**

Omega-3 supplements are generally safe for most people. However, they can cause side effects such as stomach upset, belching, fishy taste in the mouth, nausea and diarrhea.

For people with diabetes, omega-3s can help reduce the risk of cardiovascular disease, a common problem associated with diabetes. However, following the recommended dosage to minimize adverse effects is essential.

▸ **Contraindications:**

People with fish or shellfish allergies should exercise caution, as many omega-3 supplements are derived from fish oil.

▸ **Interactions:**

They can interact with anticoagulant drugs, such as warfarin, increasing the risk of bleeding. People taking these drugs must consult their doctor or pharmacist.

No direct interactions between omega-3 supplements and diabetes medications have been documented, but monitoring blood glucose levels when introducing a new supplement is always prudent.

Vitamin D

▸ **Side effects:**

It is generally safe when taken in recommended doses. However, excess vitamin D can lead to toxicity, the symptoms of which include nausea, vomiting, weakness, and elevated blood calcium levels (hypercalcemia).

For people with diabetes, maintaining adequate vitamin D levels can improve insulin sensitivity and glycemic control, but it is critical to avoid overdosing to prevent adverse effects.

▸ **Contraindications:**

People with hypercalcemia or kidney disease should use caution when taking vitamin D supplements, as they may exacerbate these conditions.

▸ **Interactions:**

It may interact with certain drugs, such as steroids (which can reduce vitamin D absorption) and cholesterol-lowering drugs (which can affect vitamin D absorption in the intestine).

Although there are no documented direct interactions between vitamin D and diabetes medications, monitoring blood glucose levels when introducing a new supplement is advisable.

Zinc

▸ **Side effects:**

Zinc supplements are generally safe when taken at recommended doses. However, high doses can cause side effects such as nausea, vomiting, loss of appetite, stomach cramps, diarrhea and headaches.

Zinc can help improve insulin sensitivity and blood sugar control in people with diabetes, but the recommended dose should not be exceeded to avoid adverse effects.

▸ **Contraindications:**

People with zinc allergies or conditions that affect mineral absorption should be cautious when taking these supplements.

> **Interactions:**

It may interact with certain antibiotics and rheumatoid arthritis medications, reducing their effectiveness. Therefore, it is advisable to take them at different times of the day.

There are no known direct interactions with diabetes medications, but monitoring blood glucose levels when introducing a new supplement is always prudent.

FOODS THAT TRANSFORM

"We are what we eat. Healthy eating is the first step toward a full and harmonious life" (Ann Wigmore)

Throughout history, our diet has undergone profoundly radical changes, sharply diverging from the habits of our ancestors. Millions of years ago, early humans shaped their diet around what they could gather or hunt, relying on fresh and raw foods provided by their environment. The emergence of agriculture and livestock farming marked the beginning of a new era of human nutrition, further accelerated by the Industrial Revolution. However, it is important to recognize that while our dietary habits have evolved drastically, our genetics have remained virtually unchanged.

Over time, foods such as dairy products, grains, refined sugars, and vegetable oils were introduced, alongside the rise of intensive meat production. These innovations have made meals more accessible and convenient, yet they have also led to significant changes in nutritional composition. Furthermore, advances in food preservation and culinary techniques gave rise to new methods of storage and preparation, which inevitably impacted food quality.

In recent years, an alarming trend has surfaced: modern diets have become dominated by ultra-processed foods, contributing to the widespread increase in chronic illnesses. Conditions such as obesity, type 2 diabetes, hypertension, and a variety of cardiovascular and digestive disorders have all been closely linked to this dietary shift. Why is this happening? Primarily because ultra-processed foods are heavily laden with refined carbohydrates, unhealthy fats, added sugars, chemical additives, and low-quality vegetable oils. Even meats and other animal products from intensive farming systems are often filled with substances harmful to health. These processed foods have largely replaced traditional diets, which were built on fresh and natural ingredients, disrupting the equilibrium that once fostered optimal well-being among our ancestors.

Nonetheless, there is hope for reversing this trend: small yet thoughtful changes to our eating habits can have a significant impact on our health. Returning to a balanced, nutrient-rich way of eating, centered on fresh, whole foods, is essential for establishing a strong foundation for wellness. Integrating fruits, vegetables, root vegetables, legumes, nuts, and seeds into the diet is a powerful step toward revitalizing the way we nourish ourselves. Despite this, one major challenge persists: the consumption of these natural, unprocessed foods remains astonishingly low in many parts of the world.

Choosing a lifestyle rooted in mindful eating not only helps prevent diseases associated with poor dietary habits but also rejuvenates the body and mind. By prioritizing real, wholesome foods and cutting back on ultra-processed options, we can cultivate a healthier, more balanced, and fulfilling life. Now is the time to rediscover the transformative power of a healthy diet—not as a form of restriction, but as an act of self-care. Your health deserves that commitment!

Understanding the Link Between Nutrition and Health

How often have you asked yourself if what you eat truly supports your well-being? The relationship between nutrition and health is far deeper than we commonly realize. Understanding which foods promote wellness and which ones to avoid, tailored to your specific needs, is a powerful step toward improving your quality of life. This isn't a new concept; it has been examined and revered for centuries. Since ancient times, cultures around the world have recognized the therapeutic value of nutrition as a means to heal, strengthen, and sustain the body, leaving us a profound legacy of wisdom.

Traditional medical systems—such as Traditional Chinese Medicine, the practices of ancient Egypt, Greece, and Rome, Ayurveda in India, and indigenous healing methods across the

Americas–delved into the restorative potential of natural foods. These practices emphasized the idea that food does much more than nourish; it can protect, alleviate discomfort, and even heal the body.

For many years, these age-old principles were often dismissed by conventional medicine as unscientific. Yet, modern research has gradually confirmed what our ancestors intuitively understood: the foods we eat directly affect not only our physical health but also our emotional well-being. Today, scientific studies continue to uncover compounds in food with therapeutic properties that help prevent diseases, reduce symptoms, and promote overall health.

Researchers have spent decades analyzing how certain foods strengthen the body and protect against chronic illnesses, identifying dietary patterns in populations with low disease rates that differ significantly from those in less healthy communities. These studies reveal the decisive role specific nutrients play in promoting vitality and longevity, with certain foods offering unique benefits such as anti-inflammatory properties to manage joint pain and chronic discomfort, antimicrobial effects to bolster immune defenses, anticoagulant actions to support cardiovascular health, antihypertensive abilities to regulate blood pressure, and mood-enhancing compounds that alleviate anxiety while fostering emotional resilience.

What you choose to eat influences not only your daily energy but also your capacity to recover, fend off illness, and pursue a fulfilling life. On the flip side, a poor diet or reliance on unhealthy foods can exacerbate health problems, intensify symptoms, and undermine overall well-being.

The encouraging part? Every day offers the chance to make dietary choices that lead to better health. While external factors like pollution or environmental changes may remain out of your control, your diet is a fundamental tool for self-care. Each ingredient on your plate carries the potential to positively impact both your physical and mental health.

Learning which foods are best for your unique needs–and

understanding which ones may harm your health–can empower you to find balance and achieve a healthier, more vibrant lifestyle. Nutrition, humanity's earliest form of medicine, is not just a pathway to wellness but also a connection to our roots, equipping us for a future filled with possibilities.

I invite you to explore how nutrition can become your strongest ally in easing ailments, building resilience, and fostering happiness. Are you ready to embrace this journey of discovery and transformation? Your well-being is within your control, and every meal is a chance to create a life of greater health and vitality. Start today: Nourish your body, refresh your mind, and live fully.

The Importance of Nutrition in Diabetes

When it comes to diabetes, proper nutrition is not just a daily habit–it's a cornerstone for maintaining health and enhancing quality of life. The primary objective of a well-designed nutritional plan is to keep blood glucose levels as close to normal as possible. This can be achieved through a balanced diet that carefully manages carbohydrate intake, as carbohydrates have the most significant impact on blood sugar levels. It's not simply about reducing them, but about learning to select the right types and consuming them in appropriate portions.

The amount and type of carbohydrates consumed must be closely monitored. Opting for complex carbohydrates–found in whole grains, legumes, and vegetables–is a far more effective strategy than consuming simple carbohydrates, such as those present in products with added sugars. This approach, coupled with proper portion control, plays a key role in managing diabetes effectively.

That said, the significance of proper nutrition in diabetes extends beyond just blood sugar regulation. A well-structured diet serves as a protective shield against serious complications associated with the disease, such as cardiovascular problems, kidney damage, and neuropathy. Furthermore, it supports weight loss or the maintenance of a healthy weight, which helps reduce the risk of developing other related conditions.

In addition, making informed food choices can lead to improved daily energy levels and a positive impact on overall mood. Feeling good isn't just about achieving favorable lab results–it's also about having the vitality to fully enjoy daily life while maintaining both physical and emotional well-being.

Questions and Answers about Food

Here are a series of frequently asked questions about diet and their answers to help you better understand how to manage your diet in case of diabetes:

1. Why is it essential for a person with diabetes to avoid foods with a high glycemic index?

Foods with a high glycemic index often cause rapid increases in blood glucose levels, making it difficult to control diabetes.

2. What is a healthy alternative to sugar-sweetened beverages?

A healthy alternative is water with lemon slices or herbal teas without sugar.

3. What beverages are safe for a person with diabetes?

The best choices include water, unsweetened tea or infusion, unsweetened coffee, and occasionally low-calorie or stevia-sweetened beverages.

4. Is it safe to consume artificial sweeteners?

Many artificial sweeteners are considered safe for people with diabetes, but they should be used in moderation and consultation with a physician or nutritionist.

5. How does excessive alcohol consumption affect a person with diabetes?

Alcohol can cause both hypoglycemia and hyperglycemia, depending on the amount and type consumed. It can also interfere with the effectiveness of diabetes medications.

6. What impact do trans fats have on people with diabetes?

Avoiding trans fats can increase the risk of inflammation,

insulin resistance and cardiovascular disease.

7. How can healthy fats benefit a person with diabetes?

Healthy fats often help improve insulin sensitivity and reduce the risk of cardiovascular disease.

8. Why is consuming whole grains preferable to refined flour?

Whole grains contain more fiber, which helps slow glucose absorption into the bloodstream, keeping sugar levels more stable and promoting better digestion.

9. How does fruit consumption affect the diet of a person with diabetes?

Fruits are an essential source of vitamins, minerals and fiber. However, to avoid blood sugar spikes, they should be consumed in moderation, preferably whole.

10. What role does fiber play in the control of diabetes?

Fiber helps regulate blood sugar levels by slowing digestion and glucose absorption, providing a feeling of satiety that helps control weight.

11. Why is it essential to control sodium intake in a person's diet with diabetes?

People with diabetes have an increased risk of hypertension. Reducing sodium intake can help control blood pressure and reduce the risk of heart disease.

12. How can portion control benefit a person with diabetes?

Portion control helps to avoid excessive consumption of calories and carbohydrates, which facilitates the management of blood sugar levels.

13. Why is it important to read food labels?

Reading labels lets you identify sugar content, saturated and trans fats, and other ingredients that could negatively affect diabetes control.

14. What is the glycemic index, and why is it essential for

people with diabetes?

The glycemic index (GI) measures how carbohydrate-containing foods affect blood glucose levels. Foods with a low GI are digested and absorbed more slowly, which helps keep glucose levels more stable.

15. How do fast foods affect people with diabetes?

Fast foods are often high in saturated fats, refined carbohydrates and sodium, which frequently cause blood glucose spikes and increase the risk of heart disease.

16. What types of protein are most recommended for people with diabetes?

Lean proteins, such as skinless chicken, fish, legumes, and tofu, are healthy choices as they have less saturated fat and provide essential nutrients.

17. Why is it essential to avoid processed foods?

Processed foods often contain added sugars, trans fats and sodium, which can complicate blood glucose control and increase the risk of complications.

18. What role does hydration play in the management of diabetes?

Staying well hydrated is crucial because it helps the kidneys eliminate excess glucose through urine and helps prevent dehydration, which can affect blood sugar levels.

19. How can a person with diabetes handle the temptations of unhealthy foods?

Planning meals, keeping healthy options on hand, not buying what you don't want to eat, and practicing portion control help manage temptations. It is also helpful to set goals and reward yourself with non-food choices.

20. What effects do complex carbohydrates have on blood glucose levels?

Complex carbohydrates, such as those found in whole grains and legumes, are digested more slowly, which helps keep blood sugar levels more stable.

21. Why is it important to include vegetables in a person's diet with diabetes?

Vegetables are low in calories and high in fiber, vitamins and minerals. They help control weight and improve overall health and blood glucose control.

22. What strategies can help a person with diabetes eat healthy meals away from home?

Some valuable strategies are choosing grilled or baked dishes instead of fried, asking for dressings and sauces on the side, opting for small portions, and choosing water or sugar-free beverages.

23. Why would combining carbohydrates with proteins and/or fats at each meal be convenient?

Combining carbohydrates with protein and/or fat at each meal is important because it helps slow the digestion and absorption of carbohydrates. This prevents rapid spikes in blood glucose, which is especially beneficial for people with diabetes, as they need to maintain stable blood sugar levels. Proteins and fats also provide a more prolonged feeling of satiety, helping to control appetite and prevent overeating. In addition, a balanced combination of macronutrients ensures that all the essential nutrients needed for energy and optimal body function are obtained.

Cooking Techniques

Healthy cooking is essential for everyone, particularly after the age of 40. Below are various cooking techniques and their related health benefits and risks.

Healthier ways of cooking

‣ **Steaming**: The steaming method is an excellent option for preserving the nutrients in food, as no additional fats are used. Steaming helps keep the food tender and juicy and is a gentle way of cooking that does not contribute to the formation of harmful compounds.

‣ **Oven roasting**: Oven roasting is a healthy cooking method that does not require added oils. Various foods, such as vegetables, fish, and chicken, can be roasted in the oven for a nutritious and tasty meal.

‣ **Light sautéing**: Light sautéing involves cooking food quickly over high heat with a healthy oil, such as olive or coconut oil. This technique allows the food to cook rapidly while preserving its texture and nutrients.

‣ **Boiling**: Boiling is a healthy way of cooking, especially for vegetables. It preserves the nutrients and produces a tender texture. However, it is essential to cook vegetables sparingly to avoid nutrient loss.

‣ **Baking**: Baking is a great way to cook food without adding extra oils. You can bake fish, poultry, vegetables, and whole grains for healthy and delicious dishes.

Less healthy ways of cooking

‣ **Frying**: Frying involves dipping food in hot oil, which increases the amount of saturated fat and calories. Additionally, frying at high temperatures generates compounds that are harmful to health.

‣ **Breading and battering**: Breading and battering food increases its calories and fat content. Breaded foods absorb more oil during cooking, resulting in a less healthy meal.

‣ **Creamy sauces and dressings**: These sauces often contain high amounts of saturated fat and extra calories, increasing inflammation and worsening pain.

‣ **Grilling at high temperatures**: Cooking food on the grill can generate harmful compounds, such as polycyclic aromatic hydrocarbons and heterocyclic amines, linked to an increased cancer risk. Additionally, grilled meat often generates inflammatory compounds.

Remember that how you cook food can impact its nutritional value and how it affects your body. It is essential to choose healthy cooking methods to maximize the benefits of food and reduce potential adverse effects.

Beneficial Foods for Diabetes

Choosing the right foods and beverages is essential for managing diabetes, as it helps maintain stable blood glucose levels and reduces the risk of long-term complications. Below, we will explore the most recommended options and their positive impact on health.

▶ **Green leafy vegetables**
Examples: Spinach, kale, chard.
Benefits: They are low in calories and carbohydrates but rich in fiber, vitamins (such as A, C, K), and minerals (such as magnesium). Fiber helps improve blood sugar control.

▶ **Healthy oils**
Examples: Olive oil and avocado oil.
Benefits: Monounsaturated and polyunsaturated fats can help reduce bad cholesterol (LDL) and improve cardiovascular health.

▶ **Lean protein**
Examples include skinless chicken, fish (especially fatty fish such as salmon and tuna), legumes, and tofu.
Benefits: Lean proteins are essential for body growth and repair and do not raise blood glucose levels.

▶ **Legumes**
Examples: Lentils, chickpeas, beans, peas.
Benefits: They are an excellent source of vegetable protein, fiber, B vitamins, iron and other minerals. Fiber helps to improve glycemic control and increase satiety.

▶ **Low-fat dairy products**
Examples: Plain yogurt, low-fat milk, low-fat cheese.
Benefits: Plain yogurt provides calcium and vitamin D, which are essential for bone health. It also contains probiotics, which benefit intestinal health.

▶ **Low glycemic index fruits**
Examples: Berries (strawberries, blueberries, raspberries, blackberries), pears, apples, and plums.
Benefits: They provide fiber, vitamins and antioxidants. Fruits

with low glycemic indexes have a lower impact on blood sugar
levels.

> **Nuts and seeds**
Examples: Almonds, walnuts, chia seeds, flax seeds.
Benefits: These foods are rich in protein, healthy fats, and fiber,
which help control blood sugar and promote cardiovascular
health.

> **Whole grains**
Examples: Oats, quinoa, brown rice, barley.
Benefits: Whole grains contain more fiber and nutrients than
refined grains. The fiber in whole grains slows the digestion and
absorption of carbohydrates, helping to maintain stable glucose
levels.

List of Beneficial Foods

Here is a carefully curated selection of foods particularly
recommended for people with diabetes, along with the health
benefits they offer:

Avocados

Because of their low carbohydrate content, rich in healthy
monounsaturated fats, avocados can improve heart health and
help maintain stable blood glucose levels.

Barley

This whole grain is rich in soluble fiber, which can help lower
blood sugar levels and improve digestive health.

Berries

Examples: Strawberries, raspberries, blueberries, and black-
berries.
Benefits: Berries are rich in antioxidants, vitamins and fiber
and have a low glycemic index, making them ideal for
maintaining stable blood sugar levels. They are also sweet and
healthy options for satisfying cravings.

Chia and flax seeds

These seeds are high in fiber and omega-3 fatty acids and can
help stabilize glucose levels and improve cardiovascular health.

Citrus

Examples: Oranges, grapefruit, lemons.
Benefits: They contain vitamin C, fiber, and antioxidants. Although they have natural sugar, their high fiber content helps moderate the impact on blood sugar.

Cruciferous vegetables

Examples: Broccoli, cauliflower, Brussels sprouts.
Benefits: They are low in carbohydrates and rich in fiber, vitamins and minerals. They also contain compounds that help reduce inflammation.

Cucumber

Cucumbers are very low in carbohydrates and calories. They are refreshing, aid in hydration, and are good sources of vitamins and antioxidants.

Dried fruit

Examples: Walnuts, almonds, pistachios.
Benefits: Rich in healthy fats, protein and fiber, nuts help control blood sugar and improve heart health.

Eggplant

Low in carbohydrates and rich in fiber, eggplant is an excellent choice for adding volume and nutrients to meals without significantly affecting glucose levels.

Garlic and onion

They have anti-inflammatory properties and help improve heart health. In addition, they can add flavor without the need for salt or fat.

Herbs and spices

Examples: Cinnamon, turmeric, ginger.
Benefits: Cinnamon, for example, helps improve insulin sensitivity and lower blood sugar levels. Spices and herbs add flavor without the need for sugar or salt.

Kale

Kale is rich in fiber, antioxidants and vitamins A, C, and K. It is an excellent addition to salads, smoothies and side dishes.

Legumes

Examples: Chickpeas, lentils, beans, or black beans.

Benefits: They are an excellent source of protein, fiber and complex carbohydrates. They help maintain stable sugar levels and are rich in nutrients such as iron and magnesium.

Lentils

Lentils have a low glycemic index and are high in protein and fiber, helping stabilize blood sugar levels.

Mushrooms

Mushrooms are low in calories and carbohydrates but are also a good source of fiber, B vitamins and antioxidants. They are versatile and can be added to a variety of recipes.

Natural Greek yogurt

Greek yogurt is rich in protein and has fewer carbohydrates than traditional yogurt. It can be a good choice for keeping sugar levels stable. Choose versions without added sugar.

Nuts and seeds

Examples: Almonds, walnuts, chia seeds, flax seeds.

Benefits: Rich in healthy fats, protein, and fiber, nuts and seeds can help improve heart health and keep glucose levels under control.

Oats

It is a good source of soluble fiber, particularly beta-glucan, which can help lower blood sugar levels and improve heart health.

Oily fish

Examples: Salmon, sardines, mackerel.

Benefits: These fish are an excellent source of omega-3 fatty acids, which are beneficial for cardiovascular health, reduce inflammation, and improve heart health.

Olives and olive oil

Both olives and olive oil are rich in healthy monounsaturated fats, which can improve cardiovascular health and help control blood glucose.

Peppers

Peppers are rich in vitamin C, antioxidants, and fiber. They are also low in calories and carbohydrates, making them a healthy choice for people with diabetes.

Pitaya or dragon fruit

Its low glycemic index helps avoid blood sugar spikes. It is also rich in fiber, which improves digestion and contributes to blood sugar control. It contains antioxidants that reduce inflammation and may improve insulin sensitivity.

Pure cocoa or dark chocolate

Rich in antioxidants and flavonoids, pure cocoa can improve insulin sensitivity. Opt for chocolate with at least 70% cocoa and consume it in moderation.

Quinoa

Quinoa is a whole grain rich in protein, fiber, and essential nutrients such as magnesium and iron. Its low glycemic index helps maintain stable blood sugar levels.

Spinach and chard

These leafy green vegetables are low in calories and carbohydrates but rich in fiber, vitamins, and essential minerals such as magnesium, which can improve insulin sensitivity.

Sweet potatoes

They are a source of complex carbohydrates and fiber, which helps maintain stable glucose levels. They are also rich in vitamin A.

Tofu and tempeh

These soy products are high in protein and low in carbohydrates, making them ideal for people seeking vegetarian or vegan alternatives to control their blood sugar levels.

Tomatoes

They are low in carbohydrates and rich in vitamin C, potassium, and antioxidants such as lycopene, which benefits cardiovascular health.

Beneficial Beverages

Below is a detailed list of recommended beverages, along with their benefits, to help you maintain good glucose control and promote healthy hydration.

Black coffee

Coffee contains antioxidants and can improve insulin sensitivity, but consuming it without sugar or high-fat creamers is essential.

Bone broth

Bone broth can be a nutritious and comforting option, low in carbohydrates and rich in minerals.

Coconut water

Although it contains natural sugar, coconut water is rich in electrolytes and can be a good choice for hydration. It should be consumed in moderation.

Ginger infusion

Ginger infusion helps reduce inflammation and improve digestion. It also helps regulate blood sugar.

Herbal infusions

Examples: Chamomile, peppermint, or rooibos infusions.
Benefits: These infusions are naturally caffeine–and sugar-free, a soothing and healthy option for staying hydrated.

Hibiscus infusion

This aromatic drink has antioxidant properties and can help reduce blood pressure. It is also naturally free of caffeine and added sugars.

Kefir

This fermented beverage is rich in probiotics, which benefit intestinal health and may help improve glycemic control.

Tea without sugar

Tea, especially green tea, contains antioxidants that can help improve insulin sensitivity and reduce the risk of heart disease.

Unsweetened almond milk

A low-carbohydrate alternative to cow's milk, ideal for those looking to reduce sugar intake and maintain a good nutritional profile.

Unsweetened vegetable milk

Examples: Almond milk and soy milk.
Benefits: These milk alternatives are low in carbohydrates and, if fortified, can be a good source of calcium and vitamin D.

Vegetable juices

Vegetable juices, especially those containing green leafy vegetables and celery, are usually nutritious and low in sugar. To control the ingredients, it is best to prepare them at home.

Water

It is essential for hydration and contains no calories, sugar, or carbohydrates.

Water with lemon

Adding lemon to water can improve the taste without adding sugar. Lemon also provides vitamin C and antioxidants.

Additional Strategies

Below are some practical and effective strategies you can adopt to complement a nutritious diet and optimize diabetes management:

▸ **Portion control:** Paying attention to portion size helps to avoid overconsumption of calories and carbohydrates, facilitating blood glucose control.

▸ **Timing of meals:** Eating regularly helps keep glucose levels stable. Following a planned meal schedule is beneficial.

▸ **Food combining:** Combining carbohydrates with protein and healthy fats at each meal helps slow sugar absorption and maintain stable glucose levels.

▸ **Carbohydrate education:** Understanding the difference between simple and complex carbohydrates and how they affect glucose levels helps make informed dietary decisions. Reducing the consumption of refined carbohydrates such as white breads, pastries and added sugars helps prevent glucose spikes.

▸ **Use of natural sweeteners:** Instead of sugar, natural sweeteners such as stevia or erythritol, which do not raise blood glucose levels, can be used.

▸ **Cooking at home:** Preparing meals at home allows you to control ingredients and portions better, contributing to better glucose management.

▸ **Adequate hydration:** Staying hydrated is vital for all bodily functions. Water is the best option for avoiding extra calories and sugars.

▸ **Nutrition labels:** Learning to read nutrition labels helps make informed decisions about processed foods' carbohydrate and sugar content.

▸ **Healthy cooking techniques:** Cooking methods such as grilling, steaming, baking, or sautéing instead of frying reduce unhealthy fats and calories.

▸ **Food diary:** Keeping a food diary helps identify patterns and triggers that affect blood sugar levels.

▸ **Information:** Staying informed about diabetes and nutrition can empower people to choose healthier food.

▸ **Regular blood sugar monitoring:** Monitoring glucose levels can provide valuable information on how different foods affect glycemic control.

▸ **Stress management:** Techniques such as meditation, yoga, mindfulness, tai chi and deep breathing help reduce stress, which often negatively impacts blood sugar levels. Practicing these techniques helps reduce stress, improve concentration and sleep, and make more conscious food choices.

▸ **Adequate sleep:** Sleeping is crucial for hormone control and glucose metabolism. Aim for 7 to 9 hours of sleep per night.

▸ **Weight control:** Maintaining a healthy weight is crucial in managing diabetes. Small weight losses often significantly impact glucose control.

▸ **Social support:** Joining support groups or online communities can provide motivation, advice, and the opportunity to share experiences with other people with diabetes.

▸ **Regular medical check-ups:** Regular visits to a health professional to monitor diabetes and adjust treatment as needed are essential for managing the condition effectively.

▸ **Regular physical activity:** Regular exercise, such as walking, swimming, or cycling, improves insulin sensitivity and helps control glucose levels. In addition to cardiovascular activities, strength training should be considered, as it can also improve insulin sensitivity and increase muscle mass.

▸ **Psychological support:** If you feel overwhelmed, consider seeking emotional or psychological support. Mental health is essential in managing diabetes.

Foods and Beverages to Avoid

Managing your diet is essential for effectively controlling diabetes and keeping blood glucose levels within a healthy range. Below is a detailed list of foods and drinks to avoid or limit, along with an explanation of why they may be harmful to people with diabetes.

▸ **Alcohol in excess**
Examples: Beer, liquors, sugary cocktails.
Reason: Alcohol can affect blood glucose levels and, in excess, increase the risk of hypoglycemia, especially if consumed on an empty stomach.

▸ **Canned fruits with added sugar**
Examples: Fruits in syrup, and candied fruits.
Reason: Added sugar increases the carbohydrate and caloric content, often leading to glucose spikes.

▸ **Fried foods and foods high in saturated fats**

Examples: French fries, fried chicken, hamburgers.

Rationale: Saturated fats often contribute to insulin resistance and increase the risk of cardiovascular disease.

‣ Refined flours

Examples: White bread, pasta, white rice.

Reason: These foods have a high glycemic index and rapidly increase blood glucose levels.

‣ Refined sugars and sweets

Examples: Cookies, cakes, candies, and chocolates with high sugar content.

Reason: These products contain simple sugars that are rapidly absorbed into the bloodstream, causing sudden spikes in glucose levels.

‣ Sugar-sweetened beverages

Examples: Soft drinks, fruit juices with added sugar, energy drinks.

Reason: Sugar-sweetened beverages provide a high amount of carbohydrates in liquid form, which tends to raise blood sugar levels quickly.

‣ Whole milk

Examples: Whole milk, fatty cheeses, sweetened yogurts.

Rationale: The saturated fat content in these products may affect insulin sensitivity and cardiovascular health.

Diabetes Support: Easy and Delicious Recipes

Explore a collection of simple, nutritious, and flavorful recipes thoughtfully crafted for people managing diabetes. These dishes are designed to help you maintain healthy blood sugar levels while bringing delicious variety to your daily meals. Eating healthy has never been this easy—nor this enjoyable!

Breakfast Options

1. **Plain unsweetened yogurt** with fresh berries (black-berries, strawberries, raspberries, or blueberries) and a walnuts

pinch.

2. Scrambled eggs with spinach and cherry tomatoes.

3. Cooked oatmeal with banana slices and a pinch of cinnamon.

4. Protein shake with spinach, unsweetened protein powder, and unsweetened almond milk.

5. Egg white omelet with spinach, peppers and mushrooms.

6. Toasted whole wheat bread with sliced avocado and tomato.

7. Berry smoothie with spinach, unsweetened protein powder and unsweetened almond milk.

8. Bowl of plain, unsweetened Greek yogurt with chia seeds and nuts.

9. Toasted whole wheat bread with low-fat cream cheese and avocado slices.

10. Egg sandwich on whole wheat bread with spinach.

11. Fresh fruit salad with a touch of cinnamon and some chopped nuts.

12. Bowl of cooked quinoa with unsweetened almond milk, cinnamon and blueberries.

13. Toasted whole wheat bread with black or red bean puree and tomato slices.

14. Oatmeal and banana pancakes (no sugar added) with plain Greek yogurt.

15. Bowl of assorted fresh fruits with a touch of lemon juice and fresh mint.

16. Avocado toast with poached egg and a pinch of pepper.

17. Bowl of unsweetened plain Greek yogurt with sunflower seeds and mango chunks.

18. Scrambled egg wrap with spinach and peppers in a whole wheat tortilla.

19. Green juice with spinach, cucumber, ginger and green apple.

20. Bowl of low-sugar whole-grain cereal with unsweetened almond milk and fresh strawberries.

21. Oatmeal pancakes with apple pieces and cinnamon, no sugar added.

22. Bowl of cottage cheese with sliced kiwi and chia seeds.

23. Whole wheat sandwich with turkey, avocado, and tomato slices.

24. Homemade whole-grain carrot and walnut muffins sweetened with stevia.

25. Bowl of cooked whole grain oatmeal with fresh peach pieces and slivered almonds.

26. Egg white omelet with spinach, mushrooms and low-fat cheese.

27. Rye toast with cottage cheese, strawberry slices, and a touch of cinnamon.

28. Protein shake with spinach, half a banana, and unsweetened almond milk.

29. Whole wheat toast with sliced avocado and poached egg.

30. Bowl of plain unsweetened yogurt with almonds and pear slices.

31. Banana and oat pancakes (no sugar added), served with fresh strawberries.

32. Bowl of cooked quinoa with unsweetened almond milk, cinnamon and blueberries.

33. Toasted whole wheat bread with mashed avocado, sliced tomato, and a squeeze of lemon.

Lunch Creations

1. Spinach salad with grilled chicken pieces, strawberries or raspberries, low-fat feta cheese and walnuts. Dress with balsamic vinaigrette.

2. Baked salmon with asparagus and cooked quinoa.

3. For turkey tacos, use whole wheat corn tortillas, lean ground turkey, peppers, onions, and avocado.

4. Chicken curry with sautéed vegetables and brown rice.

5. Chickpea salad: combines chickpeas, cucumber, tomato, red onion and bell pepper, dressed in oil, lemon, and olive oil.

6. Tuna salad: Mix canned tuna in water with cucumber, tomato, bell pepper, red onion and olives. Dress with olive oil and balsamic vinegar.

7. Grilled chicken breast with quinoa salad, avocado, tomato and cilantro.

8. Turkey Chili: Prepare a chili with lean ground turkey, beans, tomatoes, onion, bell pepper and spices. Serve with a green salad.

9. Lentil soup: Cook lentils with carrots, celery, onion and tomato. Add aromatic herbs such as thyme or rosemary.

10. Grilled salmon fillet with steamed asparagus and a portion of quinoa.

11. Chicken Wrap: Use a whole wheat tortilla and fill it with grilled chicken, lettuce, tomato, avocado and some low-fat yogurt dressing.

12. Greek chickpea salad: This salad combines chickpeas, cucumber, tomato, red onion, bell pepper, low-fat feta cheese and olives, dressed in olive oil and lemon.

13. Baked turkey with roasted sweet potatoes and steamed broccoli.

14. Salmon Salad: Mix grilled salmon, spinach, cranberries, walnuts and low-fat feta cheese. Dress with honey mustard vinaigrette.

15. Fish Tacos: Use grilled fish fillets, shredded cabbage, tomato, onion and a low-fat yogurt sauce in whole grain corn tortillas.

16. Lentil salad: Combine cooked lentils, tomato, onion, cucumber and bell pepper. Dress with a light vinaigrette based on olive oil, balsamic vinegar and fresh herbs.

17. Baked chicken breast with asparagus and roasted sweet potatoes.

18. Stir-fried tofu with vegetables: Stir-fry tofu with broccoli, carrots, bell pepper and onion in a low-sodium soy sauce mixture and ginger.

19. Chickpea salad with avocado: Mix chickpeas, avocado, tomato, red onion and cilantro. Dress with olive oil and lemon.

20. Baked fish with quinoa and sautéed spinach.

21. Chicken and avocado salad: Combine grilled chicken strips with avocado, tomato, corn, lettuce, and a light dressing of lemon and cilantro.

22. Lentil stew: Prepare a stew with lentils, carrots, celery, onion, tomato and vegetable broth.

23. Lettuce rolls with meat: Stuff lettuce leaves with lean ground beef, onion, bell pepper and spices, and serve with a side of steamed vegetables.

24. Quinoa salad with roasted vegetables: Mix cooked quinoa with roasted peppers, zucchini, eggplant and onion, and dress with olive oil and balsamic vinegar.

25. Lemon chicken with steamed broccoli and brown rice.

26. Salmon and avocado salad: Combine grilled salmon with avocado, spinach, cucumber, tomato, light yogurt and dill dressing.

27. Grilled chicken tacos: Use whole wheat corn tortillas and fill them with grilled chicken, shredded cabbage, pico de gallo, and a touch of lime.

28. Stuffed eggplants: Stuff roasted eggplants with a mixture of quinoa, bell pepper, onion, tomato and fresh herbs.

29. Chickpea salad with tuna: Combines chickpeas, canned tuna (in water), cucumber, bell pepper, red onion and parsley, dressed with olive oil and vinegar.

30. Baked fish fillet with asparagus and roasted sweet potatoes.

31. Chicken and apple salad: Mix grilled chicken chunks with apple, celery, walnuts and low-fat yogurt dressing.

32. Chicken stew with vegetables: Prepare a stew with chicken, squash, carrots, onion, tomato and low-sodium chicken broth.

33. Baked fish tacos: Baked white fish fillets with shredded cabbage, tomato, avocado and yogurt sauce are great for these tacos.

34. Quinoa salad with vegetables: Mix cooked quinoa with zucchini, bell pepper, tomato, corn and lemon cilantro dressing.

35. Grilled chicken breast with spinach salad, strawberries, almonds and balsamic dressing.

36. Prawn salad: Combine cooked prawns with avocado, tomato, cucumber, spinach leaves and lemon cilantro dressing.

37. Turkey stew: Prepare a stew with turkey, sweet potatoes, carrots, onion, tomato and low-sodium chicken broth.

38. Tofu wraps: Fill whole wheat tortillas with sautéed tofu, lettuce leaves, shredded carrots and low-fat tahini dressing.

39. Green bean and hard-boiled egg salad: Mix cooked green beans, sliced hard-boiled egg, tomato, red onion, and mustard and vinegar dressing.

40. Grilled fish with steamed asparagus and quinoa.

41. Salmon and quinoa salad: Combine grilled salmon with cooked quinoa, cucumber, tomato, spinach and lemon-dill dressing.

42. Lentil and vegetable stew: Prepare a stew with lentils, carrots, celery, onion, tomato and vegetable broth.

43. Grilled chicken wraps: Fill whole wheat corn tortillas with grilled chicken, lettuce, tomato, avocado and low-fat yogurt dressing.

Snacks

1. Celery sticks with natural peanut butter.

2. Cucumber slices with hummus.

3. A handful of almonds or walnuts.

4. Cottage cheese with apple slices.

5. Turkey rolls with lettuce leaves and mustard.

6. Apple slices with natural almond butter.

7. Cheese slices with cherry tomatoes.

8. Carrot sticks with hummus.

9. Plain Greek yogurt without sugar with a teaspoon of honey and slivered almonds.

10. Tomato slices with mozzarella and basil leaves.

11. Spinach, pineapple, and unsweetened coconut milk **smoothie.**

12. Rye toast with avocado and smoked salmon.

13. Unsweetened protein powder shake with spinach, unsweetened almond milk, and a teaspoon of almond butter.

14. Pear slices with cottage cheese.

15. Cucumber slices with smoked salmon.

16. Homemade granola bars with nuts, pumpkin seeds, and cinnamon (no sugar added).

17. Orange slices with a handful of almonds.

18. Celery sticks with low-fat cream cheese.

19. Rye toast with cottage cheese and tomato slices.

20. Ham rolls with cheese and spinach leaves.

21. Berry smoothie with spinach, unsweetened protein powder and unsweetened almond milk.

22. Homemade whole grain cereal bars with nuts and shredded coconut (no sugar added).

23. Pineapple slices with ricotta cheese sprinkled with a touch of cinnamon.

24. Whole wheat toast with nut butter and banana slices.

25. Apple slices with natural peanut butter.

26. A handful of mixed nuts and dehydrated cranberries.

27. Cucumber, tomato, and basil salad dressed with balsamic vinegar.

28. Unsweetened plain Greek yogurt with chia seeds and a pinch of vanilla.

29. Celery sticks with natural almond butter.

30. Cucumber slices with hummus.

31. A handful of almonds or walnuts.

32. Rye toast with cottage cheese and tomato slices.

Dinners Ideas

1. Baked salmon with asparagus and quinoa: Salmon is an excellent source of protein and healthy fats, and asparagus and quinoa are good choices for slow-release carbohydrates.

2. Chicken salad with avocado: Combine grilled chicken chunks with avocado, greens, tomato, cucumber, and a light lime and cilantro dressing.

3. Turkey tacos: Use whole wheat corn tortillas and fill them with lean ground turkey, lettuce, tomato, onion and a little homemade tomato sauce.

4. Grilled fish with grilled vegetables: Prepare a variety of vegetables such as grilled bell pepper, zucchini, onion and eggplant, and accompany them with a grilled fish fillet.

5. Quinoa salad with vegetables: Mix cooked quinoa with broccoli, cauliflower, peppers, onion, and a lemon and fresh herb dressing.

6. Chicken curry with vegetables: Prepare a curry with chicken breast, onion, bell pepper, carrots, zucchini and a light tomato sauce. Serve with brown rice.

7. Baked fish with spinach and strawberry salad: Bake a fish fillet with lemon, garlic and herbs, and accompany it with a fresh salad of spinach, strawberries and almonds.

8. Eggplants stuffed with quinoa and vegetables: Stuff roasted eggplants with a mixture of quinoa, tomato, onion, bell pepper and fresh herbs, and gratinate them in the oven.

9. Tofu stir-fry with broccoli and mushrooms: Stir-fry tofu with broccoli, mushrooms, carrots and onion in a low-sodium soy sauce and ginger, and serve with brown rice.

10. Greek chicken salad: This salad combines grilled chicken strips with cucumber, tomato, bell pepper, olives, low-fat feta cheese and yogurt-dill dressing.

11. Salmon and avocado salad: Combine grilled salmon with avocado, spinach, cucumber, tomato, and a light lemon and cilantro dressing.

12. Turkey stew with vegetables: Prepare a stew with turkey, squash, carrots, onion, tomato and low-sodium chicken broth.

13. Tofu and vegetable wraps: Fill whole wheat tortillas with sautéed tofu, lettuce leaves, shredded carrots and low-fat tahini dressing.

14. Green bean and hard-boiled egg salad: Mix cooked green beans, sliced hard-boiled egg, tomato, red onion, and mustard and vinegar dressing.

15. Grilled fish with steamed asparagus and quinoa.

16. Curried chicken salad: Combine grilled chicken with lettuce, spinach, apple, walnuts and a curried yogurt dressing.

17. Lentil soup with vegetables: Prepare a comforting soup with lentils, carrots, celery, onion, tomato and vegetable broth.

18. Chicken breast stuffed with spinach and low-fat cheese: Stuff chicken breasts with spinach and low-fat cheese, and bake them with a pinch of spices.

19. Chickpea salad with tuna: Mix chickpeas, canned tuna (in water), cucumber, bell pepper, red onion and parsley, dressed in olive oil and lemon.

20. Baked fish tacos with grated cabbage and yogurt sauce.

21. Salmon and quinoa salad: Combine grilled salmon with cooked quinoa, cucumber, tomato, spinach and lemon-dill dressing.

22. Lentil and vegetable stew: Prepare a stew with lentils, carrots, celery, onion, tomato and vegetable broth.

23. Grilled chicken wraps: Fill whole wheat corn tortillas with grilled chicken, lettuce, tomato, avocado and low-fat yogurt dressing.

24. Chickpea and tuna salad: Mix chickpeas, canned tuna (in water), cucumber, bell pepper, red onion and parsley, dressed in olive oil and lemon.

25. Baked chicken breast with asparagus and roasted sweet potatoes.

26. Eggplants stuffed with lean meat: Cut eggplants in half, roast them in the oven, and then stuff them with a mixture of lean ground beef, onion, bell pepper and tomato. Bake until tender.

27. Lemon chicken with asparagus: Grill or bake chicken breasts with a touch of lemon and serve them with grilled asparagus.

28. Spinach and strawberry salad: Toss fresh spinach with sliced strawberries, walnuts, low-fat feta cheese and balsamic vinaigrette dressing.

29. Grilled salmon with avocado sauce: Grill salmon fillets and serve with a creamy avocado, cilantro, and lime sauce.

30. Chickpea and spinach curry: Prepare a mild curry with chickpeas, spinach, onion, garlic, ginger, and a mixture of spices such as turmeric, cumin and coriander.

31. Chili with turkey: Prepare a chili with lean turkey, beans, tomato, peppers and spices. Serve with a sprinkling of low-fat cheddar cheese and avocado.

32. Chicken breast stuffed with spinach and feta cheese: Stuff chicken breasts with spinach and low-fat feta cheese, and roast them in the oven with a tomato and basil topping.

33. Salmon and avocado salad: Combine grilled salmon with avocado, greens, cucumber, tomato, and lemon-dill dressing.

34. Grilled shrimp tacos: Prepare tacos with grilled shrimp, shredded cabbage, low-fat yogurt sauce, cilantro and lime.

35. Chicken stew with vegetables: Cook a stew with chicken, carrots, celery, onion, tomato and low-sodium chicken broth.

36. Quinoa salad with roasted vegetables: Mix cooked quinoa with roasted vegetables such as peppers, zucchini, onion and eggplant, dressed with olive oil and lemon.

37. Turkey curry with broccoli and brown rice: Prepare a turkey stir-fry with a mild curry sauce, steamed broccoli and brown rice.

38. Avocado, tomato, and chickpea salad: This salad combines avocado, tomato, chickpeas, red onion and cilantro, dressed with olive oil and balsamic vinegar.

39. Baked fish with steamed vegetables: Bake a fish fillet with lemon and fresh herbs, and accompany it with a mixture of steamed vegetables.

40. Grilled chicken tacos with mango salsa and shredded cabbage.

41. Salmon and cucumber salad: Combine grilled salmon with cucumber slices, green leaves, cherry tomato and yogurt-dill dressing.

42. Chicken fajitas with peppers and onions: Sauté chicken strips with peppers and onions, then serve them in whole wheat tortillas with guacamole and homemade tomato sauce.

43. Chicken soup with vegetables: Prepare a soup with chicken pieces, zucchini, carrots, celery, onion and low-sodium chicken broth.

44. Sautéed tofu with vegetables and brown rice: Sauté tofu with broccoli, carrots, peppers and onion, and serve with brown rice.

45. Greek turkey salad: Combines grilled turkey strips with lettuce, tomato, cucumber, olives, low-fat feta cheese and lemon vinaigrette dressing.

46. Lentil salad with spinach and tomato: Mix cooked lentils with fresh spinach, tomato, red onion and balsamic vinaigrette dressing.

47. Baked chicken with asparagus and sweet potato: Bake chicken breasts with sweet potato slices and asparagus, seasoned with olive oil and fresh herbs.

48. Grilled salmon with avocado and quinoa salad: Accompany a grilled salmon fillet with a salad of quinoa, avocado, tomato, cucumber and lemon dressing.

49. Turkey tacos with mango salsa: Fill whole wheat corn tortillas with grilled turkey, shredded cabbage, homemade mango salsa and fresh cilantro.

50. Chickpea and spinach stew: Prepare a stew with chickpeas, spinach, onion, garlic, tomato, vegetable broth, and a pinch of cumin.

51. Chicken breast stuffed with spinach and ricotta cheese: Stuff chicken breasts with spinach, low-fat ricotta cheese, and garlic, and roast them in the oven with a tomato and basil topping.

52. Chicken salad with apple and walnuts: Mix grilled chicken pieces with sliced apple, walnuts, fresh spinach and low-fat yogurt dressing.

53. Stir-fried tofu with Asian-style vegetables: Stir-fry tofu cubes with bell peppers, carrots, broccoli, and onion in a mixture of low-sodium soy sauce, ginger and garlic.

54. Baked salmon with roasted Brussels sprouts: Bake salmon fillets with a touch of lemon and accompany them with roasted Brussels sprouts with olive oil and paprika.

55. Quinoa salad with roasted peppers and avocado: Mix cooked quinoa with roasted peppers, avocado, corn, fresh cilantro and lemon-cumin dressing.

56. Grilled turkey breast with spinach and strawberries: Grill turkey breasts and serve them with a salad of spinach, strawberries, walnuts and balsamic vinaigrette dressing.

57. Shrimp and avocado salad: Combines cooked shrimp, avocado, corn, tomato, red onion and cilantro, dressed with a bit of lime juice and olive oil.

58. Chicken enchiladas with salsa verde: Fill whole wheat corn tortillas with shredded chicken, onion, bell pepper, spinach and low-sodium salsa verde, and bake until hot.

59. Sauteed salmon with broccoli and mushrooms: Stir-fry chunks of salmon with broccoli, mushrooms and onion in a low-sodium soy sauce, ginger, and garlic mixture.

60. Lentil tacos with Mexican "pico de gallo" sauce: Fill whole wheat tortillas with cooked lentils, "pico de gallo" sauce, sliced avocado, and cilantro.

61. Lentil soup with vegetables: Prepare a comforting soup with lentils, carrots, celery, onion, spinach and low-sodium vegetable broth.

62. Grilled chicken breast with mango salad: Accompany grilled chicken breasts with a fresh mango salad, cucumber, green leaves and lemon dressing.

63. Baked fish tacos with cabbage and yogurt sauce: Bake fish fillets with a spicy topping and serve them in whole corn tortillas with shredded cabbage and low-fat yogurt sauce.

64. Quinoa salad with avocado and tomato: Mix cooked quinoa with avocado, tomato, cilantro, corn, and lemon-cumin dressing.

65. Chicken curry with mixed vegetables: Prepare a mild curry with chicken pieces, peppers, carrots, peas and light coconut milk.

66. Spinach salad with smoked salmon: Mix fresh spinach with smoked salmon, hard-boiled egg, avocado, cucumber and balsamic vinaigrette dressing.

67. Tofu stir-fry with broccoli and mushrooms: Stir-fry tofu with broccoli, mushrooms, bell peppers and onion in a mixture of low-sodium soy sauce, ginger and garlic.

68. Turkey burgers with kale salad: Prepare lean turkey burgers and serve them with a salad of kale, apple, walnuts and honey mustard dressing.

69. Chicken salad with quinoa and vegetables: This recipe combines grilled chicken with quinoa, cucumber, tomato, bell pepper, lemon and fresh herb dressing.

70. Chicken and vegetable soup with whole wheat noodles: Prepare a comforting soup with chunks of chicken, carrots, celery, onion, zucchini and whole wheat noodles.

71. Grilled fish with avocado and tomato salad: Prepare a grilled fish fillet and accompany it with a salad of avocado, tomato, red onion and cilantro, dressed in olive oil and lemon.

72. Chickpea salad with roasted vegetables: Mix cooked chickpeas with roasted vegetables such as peppers, zucchini, onion and eggplant, dressed with a lemon vinaigrette and fresh herbs.

73. Chicken curry with spinach and brown rice: Prepare a chicken curry with spinach and accompany it with brown rice.

74. Vegetable soup with turkey meatballs: Prepare a vegetable soup with lean turkey meatballs, carrots, celery, onion and low-sodium chicken broth.

75. Chicken salad with feta cheese and olives: This salad combines grilled chicken with lettuce, cucumber, tomato, low-fat feta cheese, olives and balsamic vinaigrette dressing.

76. Salmon salad with avocado and cucumber: Mix grilled salmon with avocado, cucumber, green leaves, cherry tomato and yogurt-dill dressing.

77. Baked chicken with roasted vegetables: Prepare baked chicken breasts with broccoli, carrots, peppers and onions, seasoned with olive oil, garlic and fresh herbs.

78. Turkey tacos with roasted Brussels sprouts: Fill whole wheat corn tortillas with grilled turkey, roasted Brussels sprouts, and homemade tomato sauce.

79. Greek lentil salad: This salad combines cooked lentils with cucumber, tomato, red onion, olives, low-fat feta cheese and lemon vinaigrette dressing.

80. Chicken stew with vegetables: Prepare a comforting stew with chicken pieces, zucchini, carrots, celery, onion and low-sodium chicken broth.

JUICES AND SMOOTHIES

"Fresh juices are the elixir of life, a powerful source of nutrients"
(Norman Walker)

Raw foods, often referred to as "living" foods, are an exceptional source of vitamins, minerals, fiber, trace elements, enzymes, and other vital compounds that support overall health. Incorporating these nutrient-rich foods into your daily diet not only aids in disease prevention but also alleviates symptoms of various health conditions, slows down the aging process, balances gut flora, and enhances energy levels and vitality.

While salads, whole fruits, and nuts are excellent raw food options, one of the easiest and most convenient ways to ensure regular intake is by preparing homemade juices, smoothies, and shakes. These beverages serve as a delicious and practical alternative for individuals who may not enjoy consuming fruits and vegetables directly, making it easier to include these essential nutrients in their diet.

In today's world, where ultra-processed foods and toxins have become increasingly prevalent, the need for natural, nutrient-dense foods is more crucial than ever. Raw foods play a vital role in supporting detoxification, maintaining health, and restoring balance to the body.

Many people tend to prepare their juices and smoothies using only fruits, often overlooking the incredible health benefits vegetables and leafy greens provide. Adding these to your recipes not only increases variety but also significantly boosts their nutritional value, enhancing their antioxidant, remineralizing, toning, and alkalizing properties. These qualities help maintain the body's balance, rejuvenate cells, and promote overall well-being. Additionally, vegetables and greens lower the glycemic index, improve satiety, and maximize the health benefits of these preparations.

However, it is crucial to understand that most store-bought juices are far from healthy options. These commercial products are often loaded with excessive added sugars, artificial sweeteners, preservatives, and harmful chemical additives. Furthermore, the pasteurization processes used during production strip away essential vitamins and enzymes, rendering them nutritionally deficient. The high level of refinement also removes fiber, a vital component of whole foods. In many cases, these juices contain only minimal amounts of actual fruit, making them highly processed and lacking true nutritional value.

One major concern with many juices and smoothies is their high glycemic index, which can cause blood sugar spikes, lead to weight gain, and contribute to long-term metabolic imbalances. To truly enjoy healthy and nourishing beverages, the best approach is to prepare them at home using fresh, natural, and high-quality ingredients. Homemade juices and smoothies are packed with nutrients that provide genuine benefits for your body and overall well-being.

Incorporating fresh juices made from fruits, vegetables, and leafy greens into your daily routine is an excellent practice for maintaining a healthy and energetic body. With endless combinations to explore, you can enjoy not only flavorful and refreshing options but also targeted health benefits, such as relief from conditions like arthritis, thanks to essential nutrients that support wellness. Making this a part of your everyday life can transform your health, boost your energy, and elevate your quality of life. Try it for yourself and feel the difference!

Tips for Consuming Juices and Smoothies with Diabetes

People with diabetes can enjoy juices, smoothies, or shakes, but they need to do so carefully by choosing the right time of day and the proper ingredients to avoid blood sugar spikes. Below are some key recommendations:

‣ Best Times to Consume Them

In the morning: Drinking juices or smoothies alongside a balanced breakfast is advisable. This helps you utilize energy throughout the day while avoiding unexpected blood sugar spikes.

After physical activity: Having these beverages after exercise can be beneficial since physical activity improves insulin sensitivity and helps the body process carbohydrates more effectively.

Between main meals: Use them as a snack between breakfast and lunch, or between lunch and dinner, to help maintain stable blood sugar levels and prevent dips.

‣ Choose Low-Sugar Ingredients

To ensure these drinks are both safe and healthy, select ingredients with a low glycemic index that minimally affect glucose levels. In this chapter, you will learn about the most suitable options.

‣ Combine Fiber and Protein for Better Control

Include a good source of fiber, such as chia seeds or whole oats, together with a protein source, like unsweetened Greek yogurt or plant-based protein powder. This powerful combination slows the absorption of natural sugars while helping to stabilize blood sugar levels.

‣ Portion Size and Frequency

Small portions: Limit your serving size to no more than 6-8 ounces (approximately 200 ml) per serving to avoid overloading your body with carbohydrates.

Occasional indulgence: Save juices and smoothies for occasional treats. Instead, prioritize eating fresh, whole fruits and vegetables, which are richer in fiber and better for blood sugar management.

‣ Always Monitor Your Blood Glucose

Check your blood sugar levels both before and after consuming juices or smoothies to see how your body responds. This will help you refine your ingredient choices and portion sizes for future servings.

By following these recommendations, you can safely enjoy homemade juices and smoothies on occasion without compromising your health. Remember, moderation and mindful ingredient selection are essential!

Juices: Unleash Their Power

Incorporating smoothies or shakes into your diet can be a fantastic way to boost your health. Below are some of their most significant benefits:

▸ **Compliance with Recommended Fruit and Vegetable Intake**: Smoothies and shakes offer a practical and enjoyable way to meet the daily recommendation of five servings of fruits and vegetables. They provide a diverse range of essential nutrients that support optimal health and overall well-being.

▸ **Easy Assimilation and Digestion**: As liquid meals, smoothies and shakes are gentler on the digestive system and allow for quicker nutrient absorption. They are especially beneficial for individuals with digestive sensitivities or challenges.

▸ **Vitamin and Mineral Powerhouse**: Made from fresh fruits and vegetables, smoothies and shakes are rich sources of essential vitamins and minerals that promote the proper functioning of the body.

▸ **Detoxification and Cleansing**: Ingredients like leafy greens and natural antioxidants help flush out toxins, enhance cell health, and support effective internal cleansing.

▸ **Balancing Body pH**: By incorporating alkaline foods, smoothies and shakes play a key role in stabilizing the body's pH levels, aiding disease prevention and improving overall wellness.

▸ **Reduction of Inflammation**: Anti-inflammatory additions such as turmeric, ginger, and leafy greens can help minimize inflammation, fostering better health and increased comfort.

‣ **A Balanced Meal Replacement**: When combined with protein, healthy fats, and complex carbohydrates, smoothies become a nourishing and balanced meal replacement. They provide sustained energy and promote fullness throughout the day.

‣ **Supports Weight Management**: With their low-calorie yet nutrient-dense profiles, smoothies and shakes encourage healthy eating habits. They help manage appetite and support maintaining or achieving an ideal weight.

‣ **Enhances Skin Health**: Packed with skin-friendly vitamins like A and C from fresh ingredients, smoothies and shakes contribute to hydrated, radiant, and healthy skin.

‣ **Slows Cellular Aging**: The antioxidants in smoothie ingredients combat oxidative damage, protect cells, and help maintain a youthful appearance.

‣ **Boosts Energy and Vitality**: Smoothies made with superfoods provide a steady energy boost, helping you stay active, energized, and revitalized throughout the day.

In conclusion, smoothies and shakes are a nutritious, convenient, and versatile addition to your diet. Not only do they make it easier to meet your daily fruit and vegetable intake, but they also offer a wide array of health benefits. Packed with essential nutrients, they support overall well-being–all while being refreshing, delicious, and easy to enjoy.

Homemade vs. Commercial Juices

Nowadays, identifying which foods truly benefit our health can be quite challenging. Supermarkets are overflowing with an extensive range of options, flaunting attractive packaging and clever designs that promise to be natural and healthy. While advertising and packaging often catch our attention, are we genuinely purchasing natural beverages made from fruits and vegetables? Do you know the key differences between home-made juices and industrial products? Are packaged products really as nutritious as they claim to be? Taking a few moments to carefully read ingredient labels and analyze their composition may uncover some surprising truths.

A few years ago, international regulations were established to define the standards that every fruit-based beverage must meet, specifying precise characteristics for each type of product. Below, we'll explore these distinctions and delve into the essential differences.

‣ Fruit Juice

Fruit juice is derived from fresh, chilled, or frozen fruits without undergoing any fermentation. It may contain separately extracted pulp and, in some cases, be blended with juice from various fruits. Labels are required to specify the composition in descending order, including the exact percentage of each fruit.

To prolong shelf life and eliminate the need for refrigeration, fruit juice is typically sterilized or pasteurized. Unfortunately, these processes result in significant nutrient loss, particularly impacting essential vitamins and enzymes. Moreover, the juice lacks the natural fiber found in whole fruits.

‣ Juice from Concentrates

Juice from concentrates is created by reconstituting dehydrated juice concentrates with water. Concentrates are produced by extracting natural juice through evaporation or other physical methods. During reconstitution, manufacturers may add aromas or pulp from similar fruits to partially restore flavor.

Though widely consumed, these juices suffer nutrient losses during production, including enzymes, vitamins, minerals, and the valuable fiber that characterizes natural fruit.

‣ Dehydrated or Powdered Fruit Juice

This product is manufactured by removing water from fruit to create a dry powder, which can later be rehydrated or sold in its dehydrated state. However, the dehydration process significantly diminishes its nutritional value, leading to the loss of enzymes, vitamins, minerals, and natural fiber.

‣ Fruit Nectar

Fruit nectar differs from pure juice as it is made using fruit concentrate, water, and added sugars or sweeteners. Its nutritional value is considerably lower compared to natural fruit juices due to its inclusion of artificial additives to enhance flavor, color, or shelf life.

▸ Juice-Based Drinks

These beverages typically combine various fruits but contain minimal actual fruit juice. Often, they lack the essential nutrients derived from fruits, consisting largely of water, artificial aromas, colorings, and sweeteners.

▸ Milk-Infused Juice Drinks

Milk-infused juice drinks include fruit juice, often from concentrates, in very small proportions. They are mixed with milk, water, flavorings, and other ingredients. These beverages are not considered true juices, and any nutrients present are artificially added during manufacturing to compensate for losses incurred during processing.

▸ Vegetable and/or Greens Juice

Vegetable and greens juices are extracted from vegetables using specialized industrial methods, often with added pulp or pureed ingredients. They may also blend various vegetables to create balanced or palatable flavors.

To extend shelf life and eliminate refrigeration requirements, these juices undergo pasteurization or sterilization, which unfortunately reduces essential nutrients, including vitamins and phytonutrients. Additionally, they lack the natural fiber of whole vegetables and may include preservatives, salt, or flavor enhancers that compromise their nutritional profile.

▸ Commercial Smoothies

Commercial smoothies are typically prepared by blending fruits, vegetables, and greens–often using purees or concentrates–with water, milk, plant-based beverages, or similar liquids. Their thicker texture comes from a higher proportion of pulp or fiber-rich components.

To enhance taste, appearance, and shelf life, industrial smoothies usually contain added sugars, preservatives, colorings, and flavorings that alter their natural composition. Moreover, they undergo pasteurization or thermal sterilization to allow room-temperature storage, further degrading their original nutrients and reducing their overall nutritional quality.

Advantages of Homemade Juices

After discovering what commercial products truly contain, it becomes evident that making juices at home offers numerous advantages. Here are the key benefits:

▸ **Complete Control Over Ingredients**: Preparing your own juices allows you to ensure the quality of the ingredients you use. There are no unnecessary additives, no preservatives, and –most importantly–no unpleasant surprises.

▸ **Variety and Creativity**: You have the freedom to choose your favorite fruits and vegetables, experiment with unique combinations, or incorporate fresh, seasonal produce. This not only provides a burst of delicious flavors but also boosts your intake of essential nutrients.

▸ **Authentic Aroma and Flavor**: Homemade juices retain the genuine aroma and taste of fresh fruits and vegetables. There's truly nothing like enjoying a freshly made juice packed with natural freshness.

▸ **Maximum Nutrient Retention**: Vitamins, minerals, anti-oxidants, enzymes, and other nutrients remain intact when you prepare juices at home, significantly enhancing their health benefits.

▸ **Premium Quality Ingredients**: Choosing fresh, seasonal produce at its peak ripeness ensures optimal flavor and exceptional nutritional value.

▸ **Seasonal Food Benefits**: Consuming fruits and vegetables that are in season supports sustainability, is more cost-effective, and often results in better taste and nutritional quality.

▸ **Total Customization**: Whether using a juicer or blender, you can adjust the consistency of your juice to your liking–

whether you prefer a light, clear juice or a thicker, fiber-rich option.

‣ **Kid-Friendly Option**: Homemade juices are an excellent way to incorporate fruits and vegetables into children's diets, especially for picky eaters. With creative flavors and fun presentations, you can make juices irresistible for kids.

Making juices at home provides several compelling advantages: complete control over ingredients, enhanced nutrient retention, and the flexibility to tailor your drinks to your preferences. It's also a simple yet effective way to promote healthy eating for the whole family.

Possible Adverse Effects

If you suffer from **gastritis, colitis, SIBO, irritable bowel syndrome, or constipation**, it's essential to take certain precautions when preparing smoothies or juices. Following these recommendations will help you enjoy their benefits without worsening your symptoms:

‣ **Use a juicer instead of a blender**: For digestive health conditions, it's often better to use a juicer rather than a blender when making juices. Juicing removes most of the fiber from the ingredients, resulting in a smoother liquid that is gentler on your digestive system.

‣ **Moderate your fiber intake**: Although fiber is highly beneficial for overall health, excessive consumption can lead to gas, bloating, or constipation–especially for individuals with sensitive digestion. Be mindful of the fiber content in your smoothies by limiting ingredients like fruit pulp, seeds, and whole grains.

‣ **Introduce juices gradually**: If you're unsure how your body will react, start with small portions. This enables you to monitor their effects on your digestion and adjust the recipes to suit your specific needs.

‣ **Consume juices on an empty stomach**: Drinking juices on an empty stomach can maximize nutrient absorption and aid digestion. This approach minimizes the risk of digestive discomfort and helps you fully benefit from the juice's nutrients.

▸ **Tailor recipes to your personal needs**: Everyone's digestive system is unique, and responses to certain foods can vary greatly. Pay close attention to how your body reacts after consuming juices, and adapt ingredient combinations to best support your health and well-being.

Preparation Tips

Preparing fresh juices is an easy and nutritious way to make the most of the vitamins and minerals found in fruits and vegetables. To optimize the process and ensure safety, consider the following recommendations:

▸ **Choose organic ingredients**: Whenever possible, opt for organic fruits and vegetables. They provide cleaner, pesticide-free consumption and promote a healthier lifestyle.

▸ **Wash ingredients thoroughly**: Rinse all produce carefully to remove dirt, bacteria, and chemical residues. Trim any bruised, moldy, or damaged areas to prevent contamination.

▸ **Cut ingredients into smaller pieces**: Make blending easier by chopping fruits and vegetables into smaller, manageable chunks. This helps achieve a smoother texture and shortens preparation time.

▸ **Balance ingredients with low water content**: Fruits and vegetables with low water content, such as bananas and avocados, may require pre-mixing. Start with juicier ingredients to create a liquid base, then gradually add denser items for a cohesive blend.

▸ **Peel certain fruits appropriately**: Remove citrus rinds (like those from oranges and grapefruits), as their outer layers may contain toxins. However, keep the nutrient-rich white inner layer. Peel tropical fruits, such as papayas and kiwis, especially if they are grown in regions with less stringent chemical regulations.

▸ **Discard harmful seeds**: Remove seeds from apples, as they contain trace amounts of cyanide and are unsafe to consume. On the other hand, seeds from grapes, melons, lemons, and limes are safe and offer additional health benefits.

▸ **Incorporate stems and leaves mindfully**: Many stems and leaves are nutritious, but be cautious. Avoid toxic ones, such as carrot and rhubarb leaves, which can be harmful.

▸ **Drink your juice immediately**: Freshly prepared juice is best consumed right away to minimize nutrient loss and avoid oxidation. This ensures maximum freshness and health benefits.

▸ **Remove bitter celery leaves**: Bitter celery leaves can affect the flavor of your juice. Remove them before blending the stalks to create a more balanced and enjoyable taste.

Key Recommendations

Smoothies and shakes are an excellent, healthy alternative, but to get the most out of them, it's essential to keep certain aspects in mind. Below are some key recommendations:

▸ **Moderate fruit consumption**: Fruits are a fantastic source of nutrients but also contain fructose, a natural sugar that, when consumed excessively, can impact your health. Strive for balance by moderating your fruit intake throughout the day. Additionally, avoid eating fruits at night, as the body may metabolize them less efficiently during this time.

▸ **Choose seasonal fruits**: Seasonal fruits are often more nutrient-rich, flavorful, and cost-effective. By opting for fruits in season, you can enjoy their peak freshness and nutritional benefits while saving money.

▸ **Pick compatible combinations**: Not all fruits or ingredients blend well together. Research suitable pairings to create a smoothie or shake with balanced flavors and optimal nutritional value.

‣ **Use a moderate amount of ingredients**: The simplest smoothies are often the best. Avoid overloading them with excessive ingredients, which can lead to heavy textures or digestive discomfort. Stick to recommended recipes and be mindful of proportions.

‣ **Include leafy greens and vegetables**: Incorporate leafy greens, like spinach or kale, or vegetables, such as cucumber, to lower the glycemic index and boost your drink's nutrient profile. These additions make your smoothie both healthier and more satisfying.

‣ **Use natural sweeteners in moderation**: Enjoy the natural flavors of the ingredients, but if sweetening is necessary, choose options like raw honey or pure stevia. Use them sparingly to maintain a balanced nutritional profile.

‣ **Chew your drink**: Even liquid smoothies benefit from being "chewed." This simple habit stimulates the release of digestive enzymes, helping improve nutrient absorption and reducing discomfort like bloating or indigestion.

‣ **Store properly**: For the best results, consume smoothies or shakes fresh. If storing is needed, place them in a dark, airtight container in the refrigerator, or freeze individual portions for later use.

‣ **Make them fun and personalized**: Add an enjoyable twist by freezing smoothies in molds with fun shapes–an excellent way to turn a healthy drink into a delightful treat, especially for children.

These recommendations will help you make the most of your smoothies and shakes. While the recipes provided in this book are crafted to facilitate nutrient absorption, always remember that individual needs vary. Feel free to experiment with different combinations, tailor recipes to suit your tastes, and prioritize your health and well-being. Enjoy the journey to a healthier lifestyle!

Recipes

Discover a wide range of nutritious and perfectly balanced recipes, specially crafted to support a healthy lifestyle for people with diabetes.

▸ Antioxidant green smoothie

Ingredients: 1 cup of fresh spinach, 1/2 cucumber, 1/2 green apple, 1/2 avocado, and 1 cup of water or unsweetened almond milk.

Instructions: Blend all ingredients in a blender until smooth. Serve immediately.

▸ Carrot and ginger juice

Ingredients: 3 carrots, 1/2 cucumber, 1 small piece of fresh ginger (to taste), and 1 lemon (optional).

Instructions: Blend the juice from the carrots, cucumber, and ginger. If desired, add lemon juice.

▸ Berry and yogurt smoothie

Ingredients: 1/2 cup mixed berries (strawberries, blueberries, raspberries), 1/2 cup plain unsweetened Greek yogurt, 1/2 cup water or unsweetened almond milk, and 1 teaspoon chia seeds (optional).

Instructions: Blend all ingredients until a homogeneous consistency is obtained. Enjoy chilled.

▸ Celery and lemon juice

Ingredients: 4 celery stalks, 1/2 lemon and 1/2 cup water.

Instructions: Blend celery with water, then strain the juice. Add the lemon juice before serving.

▸ Cucumber and kiwi smoothie

Ingredients: 1 cucumber, 1 peeled kiwi, 1/2 cup spinach, 1 cup water, and mint leaves (optional).

Instructions: Blend all ingredients. Serve cold.

▸ Tomato and basil juice

Ingredients: 2 ripe tomatoes, 1/2 red bell pepper, 1/4 small onion, fresh basil leaves, and 1 cup of water.

Instructions: Blend all ingredients until smooth. Serve cold.

‣ Zucchini and Apple Smoothie

Ingredients: 1/2 zucchini, 1/2 green apple, 1/2 lemon (juice), and 1 cup of water or unsweetened coconut milk.

Instructions: Mix all ingredients in a blender. Add ice if you want it cold.

‣ Beet and orange juice

Ingredients: 1 small beet, 1 small orange and 1 carrot.

Instructions: Peel the beets and the orange. Use a blender. Serve immediately.

‣ Spinach and berries smoothie

Ingredients: 1 cup fresh spinach, 1/2 cup blueberries, 1/2 cup strawberries, 1/2 cup plain unsweetened Greek yogurt, and 1 cup water or unsweetened almond milk.

Instructions: Blend all ingredients until a homogeneous mixture is obtained. Serve cold.

‣ Nopal and pineapple juice

Ingredients: 1 small, cleaned and chopped nopal, 1 slice of pineapple, 1/2 cucumber, and 1 cup of water.

Instructions: Blend all ingredients until smooth. Strain to remove any fibrous parts. Serve chilled.

‣ Avocado and lemon smoothie

Ingredients: 1/2 avocado, 1/2 lemon (juice), 1 cup spinach, 1 cup water, and some mint leaves (optional).

Instructions: Mix all ingredients in a blender. Add ice if you want it cold.

‣ Celery, apple and lemon juice

Ingredients: 3 celery stalks, 1/2 green apple, 1/2 lemon (juice), and 1 cup water.

Instructions: Blend celery and apple with water, then add lemon juice. Serve immediately.

‣ Kale and cucumber smoothie

Ingredients: 1 cup kale, 1/2 cucumber, 1/4 avocado, 1 cup unsweetened coconut water, and 1/2 lemon (juice).

Instructions: Blend all ingredients until smooth. Serve cold.

▸ Carrot and ginger juice

Ingredients: 2 medium carrots, 1 small piece of fresh ginger, 1 small green apple, and 1 cup of water.

Instructions: Peel the carrots and ginger. Blend all the ingredients. Strain the juice if you prefer a more liquid texture.

▸ Pumpkin and cinnamon smoothie

Ingredients: 1/2 cup pumpkin puree, 1/2 small banana (preferably green), 1 cup unsweetened almond milk, and 1/2 teaspoon cinnamon.

Instructions: Mix all ingredients in a blender. Serve chilled, adding ice if desired.

▸ Watermelon and mint juice

Ingredients: 1 cup diced watermelon (seeds removed), 1/2 cup lime juice, mint leaves to taste, and 1/2 cup water.

Instructions: Blend the watermelon, lime juice and water. Add the mint leaves and blend again. Serve chilled.

▸ Chia and berry smoothie

Ingredients: 1 cup blackberries or raspberries, 1 tablespoon chia seeds, 1 cup unsweetened coconut milk and 1/4 teaspoon vanilla extract.

Directions: Blend all ingredients in a blender. Let it stand for a few minutes to allow the chia seeds to hydrate and thicken the smoothie. Serve cold.

▸ Tomato and basil juice

Ingredients: 2 medium tomatoes, 1/2 cucumber, fresh basil leaves to taste, 1/2 lemon (juice), salt and pepper to taste.

Instructions: Blend all ingredients. Adjust flavor with salt and pepper. Serve cold and garnish with more basil leaves.

▸ Pear and spinach smoothie

Ingredients: 1 ripe pear, 1 cup of fresh spinach, 1/2 cup of natural yogurt without sugar, and 1/2 cup of water.

Instructions: Blend all ingredients until a homogeneous

mixture is obtained. Serve immediately.

‣ Beet and orange juice

Ingredients: 1 small beet, peeled and chopped, 1 orange (the juice), 1 small carrot, and 1 cup of water.

Instructions: Blend the beets, carrots and water. Add orange juice and mix well. Serve chilled.

‣ Turmeric and green mango smoothie

Ingredients: 1/2 green mango (less ripe to reduce sugar), 1/2 teaspoon turmeric powder, 1 cup unsweetened almond milk, and 1/4 teaspoon black pepper.

Instructions: Mix all ingredients in a blender. Serve cold.

‣ Celery and green apple juice

Ingredients: 2 celery stalks, 1 green apple, 1/2 cucumber, and the juice of 1/2 lemon.

Instructions: Blend all the ingredients. Strain the juice if you prefer a more liquid texture. Serve cold.

‣ Coconut and spinach smoothie

Ingredients: 1 cup fresh spinach, 1/2 cup unsweetened coconut milk, 1/4 avocado and 1 tablespoon unsweetened shredded coconut.

Instructions: Blend all ingredients until the mixture is smooth and creamy. Serve cold.

‣ Pomegranate and ginger juice

Ingredients: 1/2 cup of pomegranate seeds, a piece of fresh ginger, 1 cup of water, and mint leaves to taste.

Instructions: Blend the pomegranate seeds and ginger with the water. Strain the juice to remove any remaining solids. Serve chilled and garnish with mint leaves.

‣ Melon and cucumber smoothie

Ingredients: 1 cup diced cantaloupe melon, 1/2 cucumber, peeled and sliced, 1 cup unsweetened coconut water, and mint leaves to taste.

Instructions: Blend all ingredients until smooth. Serve chilled and garnish with mint leaves.

▸ Carrot and lemon juice

Ingredients: 2 large carrots, 1 lemon juice, 1/2 cup water, 1 small piece of fresh ginger.

Instructions: Blend the carrots, ginger and water. Add lemon juice and mix well. Serve chilled.

▸ Kiwi and spirulina shake

Ingredients: 2 peeled kiwis, 1/2 teaspoon spirulina powder, 1 cup unsweetened almond milk, and 1 tablespoon flax seeds.

Instructions: Blend all ingredients until a homogeneous mixture is obtained. Serve immediately.

▸ Watermelon and basil juice

Ingredients: 1 cup of diced watermelon, fresh basil leaves to taste, and 1/2 cup of water.

Instructions: Blend watermelon, basil and water. Strain if necessary to obtain a lighter texture. Serve chilled.

▸ Zucchini and green apple smoothie

Ingredients: 1/2 zucchini, peeled and chopped; 1 green apple, cored and chopped; 1 cup cold green tea without sugar; and 1/2 lemon juice.

Instructions: Blend all ingredients. Serve cold.

▸ Spinach and pineapple juice

Ingredients: 1 cup fresh spinach, 1/2 cup diced pineapple, 1/2 cucumber and 1 cup water.

Instructions: Blend all ingredients. Strain if you prefer a more liquid texture. Serve cold.

▸ Raspberry and chia smoothie

Ingredients: 1/2 cup fresh or frozen raspberries, 1 tablespoon chia seeds, 1 cup unsweetened almond milk, and 1/4 teaspoon vanilla extract.

Instructions: Blend all ingredients. Let it stand for a few minutes so the chia seeds can expand. Serve cold.

▸ Nopal and lemon juice

Ingredients: 1 small nopal, cleaned and chopped, and the juice of 1 lemon.

Instructions: Blend the nopal with the lemon juice and 1 cup of water. Strain to remove any fibrous parts. Serve cold.

‣ Blueberry and kale smoothie

Ingredients: 1/2 cup fresh or frozen blueberries, 1 cup kale without stems, 1 cup unsweetened coconut water, and 1 tablespoon flax seeds.

Instructions: Blend all ingredients until a homogeneous mixture is obtained. Serve cold.

‣ Cucumber and parsley juice

Ingredients: 1 large peeled and chopped cucumber, a handful of fresh parsley, 1 lemon juice, and 1 cup of water.

Instructions: Blend cucumber, parsley, lemon juice and water. Strain if desired. Serve chilled.

‣ Almond and cocoa milkshake

Ingredients: 1 cup unsweetened almond milk, 1 tablespoon unsweetened cocoa powder, 1/4 avocado, and 1 teaspoon vanilla extract.

Directions: Blend all ingredients in a blender until smooth and creamy. Serve immediately.

‣ Tomato and celery juice

Ingredients: 2 ripe tomatoes, 2 celery stalks, 1/2 lemon juice, salt and pepper to taste.

Instructions: Blend the tomatoes and celery with the lemon juice. Add salt and pepper. Strain if you prefer a smoother texture. Serve cold.

‣ Pear and ginger smoothie

Ingredients: 1 cored and chopped pear, 1/2 teaspoon grated fresh ginger, 1 cup fresh spinach and 1 cup water.

Instructions: Blend all ingredients until smooth. Serve cold.

‣ Beet and carrot juice

Ingredients: 1 small beet, peeled and chopped, 2 carrots, peeled and chopped, juice of 1 orange, and 1 cup of water.

Instructions: Blend the beets, carrots and water. Add orange juice and mix well. Serve cold.

‣ Green Mango and Spinach Smoothie

Ingredients: 1/2 green mango, peeled and chopped, 1 cup fresh spinach, 1/2 cucumber, peeled and chopped, and 1 cup unsweetened coconut water.

Instructions: Blend all ingredients until a homogeneous mixture is obtained. Serve immediately.

‣ Grapefruit and mint juice

Ingredients: 1 grapefruit juice, fresh mint leaves to taste, and 1 cup of water.

Instructions: Mix the grapefruit juice with the water and add the mint leaves. Stir well and serve chilled.

‣ Watermelon and basil smoothie

Ingredients: 1 cup of seeded and diced watermelon, fresh basil leaves, 1/2 lime juice, and 1/2 cup of water.

Instructions: Blend all ingredients until a homogeneous mixture is obtained. Serve well chilled.

‣ Red bell pepper and tomato juice

Ingredients: 1 seeded and chopped red bell pepper, 2 ripe tomatoes, 1/2 lemon juice, and 1 cup of water.

Instructions: Blend the bell pepper and tomatoes with the water and lemon juice. Strain if you prefer a more liquid texture. Serve cold.

‣ Strawberry and oat milkshake

Ingredients: 1/2 cup fresh or frozen strawberries, 2 tablespoons oatmeal, 1 cup unsweetened almond milk, and 1/4 teaspoon cinnamon.

Instructions: Blend all ingredients until well combined. Serve immediately.

‣ Green apple and spinach juice

Ingredients: 1 cored and chopped green apple, 1 cup of fresh spinach, 1/2 lemon juice, and 1 cup of water.

Instructions: Blend the apple and spinach with the water and lemon juice. Strain if desired. Serve cold.

To ensure these beverages are safe and healthy, opt for ingredients with a low glycemic index that have minimal impact on glucose levels. In this chapter, you will explore the best options available.

MEDICINAL PLANTS

"Nature is the wisest physician" (Hippocrates)

Since time immemorial, humanity has turned to the natural world for answers to its needs. Medicinal herbs, faithful companions on this journey, have generously shared their wisdom to ease ailments and enhance well-being. This ancient knowledge, carefully preserved through the ages, has found a renewed place in the modern world, offering a healthy and sustainable option to address today's challenges.

In a society increasingly conscious of the adverse effects of certain pharmaceutical treatments and the environmental toll of unsustainable practices, botanical remedies are experiencing a resurgence with renewed prominence. For those seeking a balanced, respectful lifestyle in harmony with the environment, these green treasures provide invaluable solutions. This revival not only reflects a growing interest in ecological approaches but also an evolution toward holistic care for both the body and the planet.

What makes these natural wonders truly extraordinary is the complexity of their compounds, capable of delivering antioxidant, anti-inflammatory, antibacterial, and antiviral properties, among others. Their potential ranges from alleviating everyday issues like sleeplessness or sluggish digestion to addressing conditions such as chronic stress or age-related ailments.

Beyond the ability to target specific concerns, these species serve as vital sources of micronutrients–vitamins, minerals, fiber, and antioxidants–that fortify the immune system and support long-term health. Incorporating them into dietary or self-care routines offers a simple, sustainable, and effective path toward illness prevention and enhanced overall wellness.

The botanical kingdom boasts remarkable diversity, featuring countless species uniquely suited to meet specific needs. Whether prepared as herbal teas, applied as balms or tinctures, or utilized in the form of essential oils, their applications are as versatile as they are effective, seamlessly fitting into various lifestyles.

More than mere remedies, these natural allies inspire us to reconnect with the world around us. Harnessing their benefits requires respect for environmental rhythms and a deeper appreciation for our planet's ecosystems. Each herb or extract serves as a tangible reminder of our connection to the living world, fostering a sense of harmony that transcends the physical and nurtures the spiritual.

In addition to their myriad health benefits, plant-based solutions stand out for their accessibility and practical versatility. Many species grow abundantly in wild habitats or can be easily cultivated in home gardens, offering an affordable, sustainable alternative. In a global context marked by economic inequalities, these wellness allies provide inclusive options to complement—or even replace—costly interventions.

Over the centuries, knowledge of these natural solutions has been carefully preserved through oral traditions and written records. This heritage, rooted in deep respect for biodiversity, has been bolstered by modern science, validating the effects of their active compounds and shedding light on their mechanisms of action. It represents a powerful synergy between tradition and innovation, broadening the therapeutic applications of these botanical marvels.

However, unlocking their full potential requires responsible use. Every human body is unique, and while these species possess well-documented therapeutic properties, they are not without risks. Misuse or interactions with conventional medications can lead to adverse effects. Therefore, obtaining accurate and reliable information is essential to ensure safe and effective usage.

One particularly fascinating aspect is how the components within a plant work in unison. Whole extracts, resulting from this intricate interaction, often produce more balanced and holistic effects compared to isolated compounds. Molecules interact in complementary ways, maximizing benefits while reducing potential side effects. Conversely, isolated active principles can provide concentrated solutions but may carry an increased risk of adverse effects on the body.

The innate harmony of these botanical wonders highlights one of biodiversity's greatest gifts–balance. Whole extracts are celebrated for their gentleness and ability to integrate seamlessly with the body's natural processes. On the other hand, synthesized compounds strive for potency, often at the expense of stability. The synergistic interaction between molecular components amplifies therapeutic benefits while limiting potential downsides, making them a choice deeply aligned with human needs.

Ultimately, medicinal plants transcend their role as therapeutic tools–they bridge ancestral wisdom and scientific innovation. They remind us that the health of our bodies and the well-being of our planet are profoundly interconnected. By safeguarding this invaluable legacy, we nurture not only our own health but also that of future generations, renewing the delicate balance between humanity and nature.

Essential Information

Although plants are natural in origin, they should not be considered entirely harmless. Their active compounds may cause adverse effects or trigger allergies in certain individuals.

Occasional consumption of an infusion is unlikely to cause harm. However, excessive, prolonged, or frequent use may result in discomfort, allergic reactions, or even toxicity.

Tolerance to natural remedies varies greatly among people. If you are pregnant, breastfeeding, or managing conditions such as chronic illnesses, allergies, kidney or liver insufficiency, cancer, or undergoing medical treatment, it is crucial to refer to the section titled **"Learn Everything You Need to Know About the Plants"** before using them. This section provides essential information on potential risks, contraindications, and interactions, enabling you to make informed and responsible decisions.

Guidelines for Care with Herbal Remedies

For best results, continue using the remedies until your symptoms have completely disappeared. The treatment duration will vary depending on factors like the severity of your condition, how it progresses, your personal commitment, and other important influences.

Keep in mind that some plants or herbal remedies are not suited for continuous or long-term use. In such cases, you will always find specific instructions that address this.

While following the guidelines for the remedies below, it is just as important to focus on the underlying causes of your symptoms. To better understand the root of your health concerns, I recommend referring to the first chapter of this book, specifically the section titled "Causes," where you'll discover essential insights into tackling the problem at its source.

Finally, remember that patience is vital. A condition that has lingered for months or years cannot be resolved in just a few days. Stay committed, persevere, and always prioritize your health and well-being.

Measurements

To achieve the best results when preparing infusions, decoctions, or other plant-based recipes, it is essential to follow these dosage guidelines:

- A tablespoon refers to a level tablespoon.
- A teaspoon refers to a level teaspoon.

Effective Plants for Managing Diabetes

For those managing diabetes, various natural alternatives can provide significant support. Medicinal plants have been used for centuries due to their beneficial properties, and today, some stand out for their ability to help regulate blood glucose levels. Among the most effective options are the following, listed alphabetically: **aloe vera, cinnamon, turmeric, fenugreek, gymnema, ginseng, ginger, mango leaves, bitter melon leaves, and neem.**

The ideal way to consume these plants is as infusions, decoctions, or natural blends, while avoiding sweeteners whenever possible. If you need to sweeten your drink, opt for 100% natural stevia. Stevia does not impact blood sugar levels and is safe for those with diabetes.

If you decide to take a break from using one of these plants, there's no need to worry. You can easily substitute it with another option from the list without losing their beneficial effects. Additionally, rotating between different plants allows you to follow the rest periods often recommended with herbal remedies, ensuring sustained effectiveness and preventing the body from developing tolerance.

The benefits, preparation methods, recommended doses, and maximum usage durations for each plant are carefully outlined. Furthermore, the scientific names of the plants are included in parentheses, as common names may vary by region or country.

Incorporating these plants into your routine can be an excellent complement to diabetes treatment. However, always consult your doctor before adding any supplement or medicinal plant to your regimen, particularly if you are already taking medication to manage your condition.

Aloe Vera (Aloe barbadensis)

▸ **Benefits:**
Aloe vera helps reduce blood sugar levels and improve insulin sensitivity.

▸ **Infusion/Decoction:**
Ingredients: One fresh aloe vera leaf.
Preparation: Extract the gel from an aloe vera leaf and mix it

with hot water. Let stand 5-10 minutes before consumption.

▸ **Dosage:**
Consume one cup a day.

▸ **Best time to take:**
In the morning, on an empty stomach.

▸ **Maximum time of continuous use:**
3 months, followed by a one-month break.

Bitter melon (leaves) (Momordica charantia)

▸ **Benefits:**
Bitter melon leaves help reduce blood glucose levels.

▸ **Infusion/Decoction:**
Ingredients: 5-7 fresh bitter melon leaves, or 2-3 dried leaves.
Preparation: Boil the leaves in water for 10 minutes and strain before consumption.

▸ **Dosage:**
One cup a day.

▸ **Best time to take:**
In the morning, on an empty stomach.

▸ **Maximum time of continuous use:**
2 months, followed by a one-month break.

Cinnamon (Cinnamomum verum)

▸ **Benefits:**
Cinnamon helps to improve blood glucose levels and increase insulin sensitivity.

▸ **Infusion/Decoction:**
Ingredients: 1-2 cinnamon sticks.
Preparation: Boil the cinnamon sticks in water for 10 minutes. Strain before drinking.

▶ **Dosage:**
Take one cup a day.

▶ **Best time to take:**
After meals.

▶ **Maximum time of continuous use:**
6 weeks, followed by a break of 1 to 2 weeks.

Fenugreek (Trigonella foenumgraecum)

▶ **Benefits:**
Fenugreek helps lower blood sugar levels and improve glucose tolerance.

▶ **Infusion/Decoction:**
Ingredients: 1 tablespoon of fenugreek seeds.
Preparation: Soak the seeds in water overnight and consume the next day.

▶ **Dosage:**
One cup a day.

▶ **Best time to take:**
In the morning, on an empty stomach.

▶ **Maximum time of continuous use:**
3 months, followed by a one-month break.

Ginger (Zingiber officinale)

▶ **Benefits:**
Ginger helps improve blood sugar regulation and has anti-inflammatory properties.

▶ **Infusion/Decoction:**
Ingredients: 4 thin slices (1 or 2 mm) of fresh ginger root.
Preparation: Boil in water for 10 minutes. Strain before drinking.

▶ **Dosage:**

One cup a day.

▸ Best time to take:
At any time of the day, preferably before meals.

▸ Maximum time of continuous use:
3 months, followed by a one-month break.

Ginseng (Panax ginseng)

▸ BenΩefits:
Ginseng helps to improve insulin sensitivity and lower blood glucose levels.

▸ Infusion/Decoction:
Ingredients: 4 thin slices (1 or 2 mm) of ginseng root.
Preparation: Boil the slices in water for 10-15 minutes. Strain before consumption.

▸ Dosage:
One cup a day.

▸ Best time to take:
In the morning, on an empty stomach.

▸ Maximum time of continuous use:
2 months, followed by a one-month break.

Gymnema (Gymnema Sylvestre)

▸ Benefits:
Gymnema helps to reduce glucose absorption in the intestine and increase insulin production.

▸ Infusion/Decoction:
Ingredients: 1 teaspoon of dried Gymnema leaves, 1 cup of water.
Preparation: Boil water, add the leaves, and let stand for 10 minutes. Strain and drink.

▸ Dosage:

1 cup of infusion 1-2 times a day.

> **Best time to take:**
Before meals.

> **Maximum time of continuous use:**
Continuous use for up to 3 months, followed by a one-month break.

Mango (leaves) (Mangifera indica)

> **Benefits:**
Mango leaves help improve blood glucose regulation.

> **Infusion/Decoction:**
Ingredients: 10-15 fresh mango leaves, or 5-7 dried leaves.
Preparation: Boil in water for 15 minutes. Let it stand and strain.

> **Dosage:**
One cup a day.

> **Best time to take:**
In the morning, on an empty stomach.

> **Maximum time of continuous use:**
2 months, followed by a one-month break.

Neem (Azadirachta indica)

> **Benefits:**
Neem has properties that help control blood sugar levels.

> **Infusion/Decoction:**
Ingredients: 8-10 fresh neem leaves, or 4-5 dried leaves.
Preparation: Boil the leaves in water for 5-10 minutes. Strain before drinking.

> **Dosage:**
One cup a day.

‣ **Best time to take:**
In the morning, on an empty stomach.

‣ **Maximum time of continuous use:**
3 months, followed by a one-month break.

Turmeric (Curcuma longa)

‣ **Benefits:**
Turmeric has anti-inflammatory and antioxidant properties, which help improve insulin resistance.

‣ **Infusion/Decoction:**
Ingredients: 1 teaspoon of turmeric powder.
Preparation: Mix with hot water and let stand for 5 minutes.

‣ **Dosage:**
Drink one cup a day.

‣ **Best time to take:**
With meals.

‣ **Maximum time of continuous use:**
2 months, followed by a one-month break.

Phytotherapy Recipes

Although the plants mentioned above are effective when used individually, their properties can be further enhanced when combined properly. Below are some particularly effective combinations.

‣ **Phytotherapy Recipe No. 1**
Cinnamon, Ginger, and Clove Infusion

Ingredients: 1 cinnamon stick, 1 small piece of fresh ginger (about 2 cm), 3 cloves, and 500 ml of water.
Instructions: In a saucepan, bring the water to a boil. Add the cinnamon stick, peeled ginger, and cloves. Simmer for 10 minutes. Strain the mixture and drink one cup in the morning and one in the afternoon.

Benefits: Cinnamon and ginger help improve insulin sensitivity and lower blood sugar levels.

▸ Phytotherapy Recipe No. 2
Cactus, Aloe Vera and Lemon Smoothie

Ingredients: 1 small nopal (without thorns), 1 tablespoon of aloe vera gel, 1 lemon juice, and 1 glass of water.

Instructions: Wash and cut the nopal cactus into small pieces. Mix the nopal, aloe vera gel, lemon juice, and water in a blender. Process until you obtain a homogeneous smoothie. Drink on an empty stomach.

Benefits: Nopal cactus helps reduce blood sugar levels, while aloe vera and lemon have antioxidant and anti-inflammatory effects.

▸ Phytotherapy Recipe No. 3
Eucalyptus, Sage, and Rosemary Infusion

Ingredients: 5 eucalyptus leaves, 1 teaspoon of dried sage leaves, 1 teaspoon of dried rosemary leaves, and 500 ml of water.

Instructions: Bring the water to a boil and add the eucalyptus, sage and rosemary leaves. Let it simmer for 10 minutes. Strain the infusion and drink it throughout the day.

Benefits: Eucalyptus and rosemary help improve circulation, and sage helps regulate glucose levels.

▸ Phytotherapy Recipe No. 4
Green Tea, Stevia, and Fenugreek Infusion

Ingredients: 1 teaspoon of green tea leaves, 1 teaspoon of stevia leaf or powder, 1 teaspoon of fenugreek seeds, and 500 ml of water.

Instructions: Boil water and add green tea and fenugreek seeds. Let steep for 5 minutes. Add stevia and strain the infusion. Drink a cup in the morning and another in the afternoon.

Benefits: Green tea contains antioxidants that help improve insulin sensitivity, fenugreek helps control sugar levels, and stevia is a natural sweetener that does not affect glucose levels.

▸ Phytotherapy Recipe No. 5
Ginseng, Dandelion and Mint Infusion

Ingredients: 1 teaspoon of dried ginseng root, 1 teaspoon of dried dandelion leaves, 1 teaspoon of mint leaves, and 500 ml of water.

Instructions: Bring the water to a boil and add the ginseng, dandelion and mint. Let it simmer for 10 minutes. Strain the infusion and drink it throughout the day.

Benefits: Ginseng helps improve insulin sensitivity, dandelion supports liver function, and peppermint provides a refreshing taste.

▸ Phytotherapy Recipe No. 6
Mango, Basil & Neem Leaf Tea

Ingredients: 5 mango leaves, 3 basil leaves, 3 neem leaves, and 500 ml of water.

Instructions: Wash the leaves well. Boil the water and add the leaves. Let it simmer for 15 minutes. Strain and drink on an empty stomach.

Benefits: Mango and neem leaves are known for their hypoglycemic properties, and basil helps regulate blood sugar.

Learn Everything You Need to Know About the Plants

In this section, we will explore in depth the plants recommended for treating the pathology we are dealing with. You will find information on adverse effects and interactions, as well as detailed information about each plant. From a complete description to details about their habitat, the parts used, the chemical components, their history, and the various therapeutic properties they have, this book will immerse you in a journey of discovery to get to know these wonderful plants in depth.

I aim to provide a comprehensive overview of these botanical species so you can understand their context and appreciate their potential. You will learn about their historical origin and their importance in traditional medicine.

I want you to become an expert connoisseur of these plants, able to make informed decisions in your search for relief and wellness. Get ready to broaden your horizons and discover nature's healing potential!

Aloe Vera (Aloe barbadensis)

Description:
Aloe vera, also known as aloe vera, is a perennial succulent plant in the lily family. Its leaves are fleshy and lanceolate and grow in a rosette.

Habitat and cultivation:
It thrives in warm, dry climates, preferably between 20 and 30 degrees Celsius. It requires well-drained soils and does not tolerate excess moisture. It reproduces through leaf cuttings and can be grown in pots or gardens.

Parts used:
The main parts used are the leaves, which contain a transparent gel inside. Fresh leaves are obtained by cutting and opening them. Dried leaves and the yellow sap under the leaf skin are also occasionally used.

Components:
Aloe gel contains polysaccharides, vitamins (C and E), minerals (calcium, magnesium and zinc), amino acids, enzymes and antioxidants.

History and tradition:
It has a long history of use. In ancient Egypt, it was known as "the plant of immortality." It has also been used in traditional Chinese and Ayurvedic medicine. Over the centuries, its reputation as a medicinal plant has spread worldwide.

Therapeutic properties:
Aloe vera juice is used to treat burns, wounds, insect bites, and skin conditions such as psoriasis and acne. It has also been used to relieve skin irritation and inflammation. Consumption of Aloe vera juice is associated with digestive health benefits,

relieving constipation and promoting intestinal health.

Curiosities:
It is said that Cleopatra used Aloe vera gel as part of her beauty routine. In addition, it is said that in World War II, the gel was used as a blood substitute in emergencies, as its chemical composition resembles that of blood plasma.

Side effects:
Although generally safe for topical use and moderate oral consumption, some individuals may experience adverse effects. Some people may have allergic reactions or skin irritation when applying Aloe vera gel. In rare cases, excessive consumption of Aloe juice may cause diarrhea, abdominal cramps and electrolyte imbalances. In addition, prolonged use of high concentrations of Aloe vera on the skin may cause dryness and flaking.

Contraindications:
It is not recommended for topical use on deep wounds, severe burns, or open surgical wounds, as it may delay healing. In addition, pregnant and breastfeeding women should consult a health professional before using Aloe vera products, as insufficient studies support its safety in these cases.

Interactions:
It may increase the risk of bleeding in people taking anticoagulant drugs. It may also interfere with the absorption of oral medications, such as angiotensin-converting enzyme inhibitors used to treat high blood pressure.

Bitter melon (Momordica charantia)

Description:
Bitter melon is a climbing plant of the Cucurbitaceae family native to Africa and tropical Asia. It is characterized by its elongated, rough, light green to dark green fruits, which have protuberances that give them a unique appearance. The leaves are large, lobed, and toothed, and the flowers are yellow.

Habitat and cultivation:
It prefers warm, humid climates and is grown worldwide in tropical and subtropical regions. To grow optimally, it needs well-drained soils rich in organic matter. As a climbing plant that requires support, it can be grown in gardens, orchards, or pots. It is a hardy and productive plant that can provide fruits throughout the year in suitable climates.

Parts used:
The most used parts are the unripe fruits, leaves and seeds. The fruits are the most well-known and appreciated for their bitter taste and medicinal properties. The leaves and seeds also contain beneficial compounds that can be used to prepare infusions, extracts, or tinctures.

Components:
It contains charantin, momordicin, polyphenols, flavonoids, alkaloids and terpenoids.

History and tradition:
For centuries, it has been used in traditional medicine in Asia and Africa for its medicinal properties. In Ayurvedic medicine, it is considered a bitter plant that balances the "doshas" and is used to treat digestive disorders, skin problems, diabetes and inflammatory diseases. In traditional Chinese medicine, it promotes blood circulation, reduces fever, and relieves pain.

Therapeutic properties:
It has hypoglycemic, hepatoprotective, antioxidant, anti-inflammatory, antimicrobial, and anticancer properties. It is used to control blood sugar levels in people with diabetes, improve liver function, strengthen the immune system, reduce inflammation, prevent infections, and protect against cancer. It has also been used to promote weight loss and improve digestion.

Curiosities:
In some countries, it is consumed as a food and prepared in various ways, such as salads, stews, or juices.

Traditional medicine uses it to treat various conditions, from digestive problems to diabetes and cancer.

It is a hardy plant that can grow in adverse conditions.

Side effects:
Excessive consumption may cause stomach upset, diarrhea, nausea, or hypoglycemia in some people.

Supplements or concentrated extracts may increase the risk of side effects. Therefore, it is essential to consume them in moderation and watch for any signs of discomfort after ingestion.

Contraindications:
It is not recommended for people with known allergies to plants of the Cucurbitaceae family, such as cucumber or pumpkin, as it may trigger allergic reactions.

Pregnant or lactating women should avoid its consumption.

Interactions:
It may interact with hypoglycemic drugs, blood pressure drugs, anticoagulants, or anti-inflammatory drugs, which may increase or decrease their effects. Consult your doctor or pharmacist.

Cinnamon (Cinnamomum verum)

Description:
Cinnamon is an aromatic and flavorful spice obtained from the inner bark of Cinnamomum trees. Several species of cinnamon trees exist, but the most common ones are Cinnamomum verum and Cinnamomum cassia. Cinnamon has a distinctive sweet odor and a warm, slightly spicy flavor.

Habitat and cultivation:
Cinnamon is native to Sri Lanka but is also cultivated in other tropical regions of Asia, such as Indonesia, India and Vietnam. It prefers warm, humid climates and is usually found at low to medium altitudes. To thrive, cinnamon trees need well-drained, nutrient-rich soils.

Parts used:
The part used is its inner bark. To obtain it, the bark is peeled from the young branches of the cinnamon tree. The bark is extracted in thin strips that are then rolled to form what we know as cinnamon sticks. Cinnamon can also be found in powdered form, obtained by grinding dried cinnamon sticks.

Components:
The most prominent compounds are essential oils, such as cinnamaldehyde, which gives cinnamon its distinctive aroma. The oil also contains eugenol, linalool and coumarin.

History and tradition:
Cinnamon has been appreciated for centuries. In ancient times, it was used as a spice, perfume and medicine. It was considered a treasure and was used in religious rituals and embalming practices. During the Middle Ages, it was a highly valued spice in Europe, and it was one of the drivers of exploration and trade in search of new routes to cinnamon-producing regions.

Therapeutic properties:
It has antioxidant, anti-inflammatory, and antimicrobial properties. It has also been studied for its effects in regulating blood sugar and improving insulin sensitivity, which benefits people with type 2 diabetes. In addition, it helps reduce LDL cholesterol, improve digestion, and relieve stomach upset.

Curiosities:
It should be noted that cinnamon has been used historically as an aphrodisiac. Its aroma and flavor are said to awaken sexual desire. In addition, cinnamon has been considered a valuable spice and used as a currency of exchange in some ancient cultures.

It has been traditionally used as an insect repellent. Its strong, spicy aroma helps keep mosquitoes and other pesky insects away. It can even be used as an essential oil to repel insects naturally.

Side effects:

It has been observed that excessive consumption can irritate the mouth and digestive tract. This is due to its content of compounds such as cinnamaldehyde, which can irritate in high concentrations.

In addition, some people may experience allergic reactions, such as skin rashes or difficulty breathing.
A potentially dangerous side effect of cinnamon is its coumarin content. Coumarin is a compound that can be toxic to the liver in high doses. However, the amount of coumarin varies depending on the species and how it is processed. Ceylon cinnamon (Cinnamomum verum) has lower levels of coumarin than cassia cinnamon (Cinnamomum cassia), which is more commonly found in the market.

Contraindications:
It is recommended to avoid its consumption in large quantities during pregnancy, as it may stimulate the uterus and increase the risk of miscarriage. In addition, people with liver disease or coagulation disorders should be cautious when consuming it, as it may affect liver function and increase the risk of bleeding.

Interactions:
It is important to note that it may interact with some medications used to treat diabetes. It can potentiate the effects of these drugs and decrease blood sugar levels, which can lead to hypoglycemia. Therefore, monitoring blood sugar levels and adjusting drug dosage in consultation with a physician is crucial.

Dandelion (Taraxacum officinale)

Description:
Dandelion is a perennial herbaceous plant in the Asteraceae family. It is medium-sized and can grow to 30 to 40 centimeters in height. Its toothed leaves form a basal rosette at the base of the plant. The plant's bright yellow flowers are grouped in characteristic heads resembling tiny suns. After flowering, the flowers give way to a fluffy white seed head, easily dispersed by the wind.

Parts used:
Both leaves and roots are used for medicinal purposes. The young and tender leaves can be used in salads or cooked as vegetables. The roots are dried and used to make infusions, extracts and tinctures.

Components:
The leaves contain vitamins A, C, and K and minerals such as iron, calcium and potassium. The roots contain inulin, a type of soluble fiber, phenolic compounds, flavonoids and triterpenoids.

History and tradition:
Dandelion seeds have been used in traditional medicine for centuries. Their use dates back to ancient Greece and Rome, where they were used to treat digestive and liver problems. They are also used in traditional Chinese and Ayurvedic medicine. In addition to their medicinal properties, dandelion seeds have a place in cultural tradition. For example, in some European cultures, blowing dandelion seeds is believed to bring good luck or fulfill wishes.

Therapeutic properties:
It has traditionally been used to stimulate digestion, relieve bloating and constipation, and promote liver and gallbladder health. Its diuretic properties help eliminate fluids and toxins from the body. It has also been used to manage diabetes, promote kidney health, and improve kidney function. In addition, it has antioxidant and anti-inflammatory properties, making it helpful in treating inflammatory conditions.

Curiosities:
Its name comes from the French "dent de lion". This is due to the shape of its leaves, which resemble the teeth of a lion. Another curiosity is that all plant parts are edible and have health benefits. Every part, from the flowers to the roots, can be used in cooking or natural medicine. In addition, it is one of the first plants to bloom in spring, and its bright yellow flowers are a sign that winter is over and the growing season is in full swing.

Side effects:
Although it is generally safe for most people, it may cause

some adverse effects. The most common symptoms include stomach upset, diarrhea, and allergic reactions in sensitive individuals. In addition, because it is a diuretic, it may increase urine output. This may benefit some people, but can also lead to dehydration if insufficient fluid is consumed.

Contraindications:
Although dandelion is considered safe for most people, there are some contraindications. People with known allergies to plants in the Asteraceae family, such as ragweed, chrysanthemum, or daisy, should avoid consuming them. In addition, people with bile duct obstruction or gallstones should avoid it, as it may increase bile production and worsen these problems.

Interactions:
It may increase the effects of diuretic drugs, which may result in increased removal of fluids and electrolytes from the body. In addition, it may interact with medications that are metabolized in the liver, such as blood thinners, diabetes and cholesterol medications. If you are taking medication, consult your doctor or pharmacist.

Eucalyptus (Eucalyptus)

Description:
Eucalyptus is a genus of trees and shrubs belonging to the Myrtaceae family, with more than 700 species, Eucalyptus globulus being one of the best known. They are fast-growing trees known for their great height, which can exceed 60 meters in some species. They have a straight, elongated trunk with bark that can be smooth, peeled in strips, rough, or persistent. The leaves are elongated, bluish-green, and give off a characteristic aroma due to the essential oil they contain. The small flowers are grouped in umbels, producing a woody fruit called a capsule.

Habitat and cultivation:
It is native to Australia and Tasmania and forms a fundamental part of the local ecosystem. However, due to its adaptability and rapid growth, it has been introduced to many other parts of the world, including South America, Africa, Asia and the Mediterra-

nean. They thrive in a variety of soils but prefer well-drained, sunny soils. They are widely cultivated for timber, paper and essential oil production. However, their cultivation has been controversial due to their environmental impact, such as depletion of water resources and reduction of local biodiversity.

Parts used:

The most commonly used parts are the leaves, from which the essential oil is extracted. This oil is the primary source of its use in natural medicine. The bark and trunk are also used in the wood and paper industry.

Components:

The most prominent component is the essential oil, which contains cineol (eucalyptol) as the main active compound. This oil also contains other elements such as limonene, pinene and flavonoids. The leaves are rich in tannins and other antioxidant compounds that contribute to their medicinal properties.

History and tradition:

Its use dates back to the traditional practices of indigenous Australian peoples, who used the leaves to treat wounds and respiratory diseases. With European colonization, eucalyptus was introduced to other parts of the world, and its essential oil gained popularity as a natural remedy. In the 19th century, European physicians recommended it to treat respiratory infections and as a disinfectant. Its wood has also been valuable in the construction and papermaking industries.

Therapeutic properties:

It is widely recognized for its therapeutic properties and is used in various applications of natural medicine:

Antiseptic and antimicrobial properties: Its oil has strong antimicrobial properties, which make it effective in cleaning wounds and disinfecting surfaces.

Improves respiratory conditions: It is popular for treating respiratory conditions such as asthma, bronchitis, and colds. It helps clear the airways and acts as an expectorant to relieve coughs.

Anti-inflammatory and analgesic properties: It is used topically to relieve muscle and joint pain, thanks to its ability to reduce inflammation and pain.

Mental stimulant: Inhaling the aroma helps to improve concentration and reduce mental fatigue.

Insect repellent: Its essential oil is used as a natural insect repellent, effective against mosquitoes and other flying insects.

Curiosities:
Koalas and eucalyptus trees: Eucalyptus trees are famous for being the primary food source for koalas, a marsupial native to Australia. Although there are many species of eucalyptus, koalas are selective and only consume certain varieties that meet their nutritional needs.

Fast growth: They are known for their rapid growth. Some species can reach heights of up to 2 meters in one year, which makes them ideal for the timber and paper industry.

Influence on climate: Eucalyptus forests in Australia are known to create a bluish haze in the air. This phenomenon is caused by the release of volatile compounds from the oil in their leaves, which scatter sunlight.

Historical use in medicine: In the 19th century, the leaves were used to purify the air in hospitals due to their antiseptic properties. Their ability to fight pathogens made them valuable during infectious disease outbreaks.

Adverse or side effects:
Its use may cause adverse effects in some circumstances:

Skin irritation: The essential oil is powerful and may cause irritation or contact dermatitis if applied directly to the skin without dilution.

Respiratory problems: Inhaling large amounts of eucalyptus oil may irritate the respiratory tract, especially in people with asthma or allergies.

Allergic reactions: Some people may experience allergic reactions, including skin rashes, difficulty breathing, or swelling.

Contraindications:
Young children: Essential oil use is not recommended for infants or young children, as it may cause severe respiratory problems.

Pregnancy and breastfeeding: Pregnant or breastfeeding women should avoid the use of essential oils due to the lack of evidence on their safety in these stages.

Pre-existing medical conditions: People with liver or kidney disease should avoid excessive use, as it may affect drug metabolism in the liver.

Interactions:
Anti-diabetic drugs: Eucalyptus lowers blood sugar levels, so people taking diabetes medications should use it cautiously to avoid hypoglycemia.

Anesthetics: It may interfere with anesthesia during surgical procedures. It is recommended that its use be suspended before surgery.

Other essential oils: Mixing eucalyptus oil with other essential oils can enhance or alter their effects, so it is vital to know each one's properties before combining them.

Fenugreek (Trigonella foenumgraecum)

Description:
Fenugreek is an annual herbaceous plant belonging to the Fabaceae family. It is native to the Mediterranean region but is now cultivated in many parts of the world. It has erect, branched stems, trifoliate leaves, and small white or pale yellow flowers. The seeds are small and oval-shaped, with a light brown color.

Habitat and cultivation:
Fenugreek can be found in a wide variety of habitats, from

coastal to mountainous. It prefers well-drained, fertile soils and can grow in full sun or partial shade. This hardy plant can tolerate adverse conditions like drought and poor soil. Fenugreek is grown mainly for its seeds, which are used for culinary and medicinal purposes.

Parts used:
The seeds and leaves are used for medicinal and culinary purposes. The seeds can be used whole or ground, while the leaves can be consumed fresh or dried.

Components:
The seeds are rich in protein, dietary fiber, minerals such as iron, calcium, and magnesium, and B vitamins. They also contain saponins, flavonoids, phytosterols, anti-inflammatory and antioxidant compounds. The leaves also contain nutrients such as iron, calcium and vitamin C.

History and tradition:
Ayurvedic medicine has a long history of use in traditional medicine. In India, it treats various conditions, such as indigestion, diabetes and respiratory problems. In addition, it promotes breastfeeding and is an aphrodisiac in traditional Chinese and Arabic medicine. It is also used in the cuisine of many cultures, especially in Indian cuisine, where it is added to curries and lentil dishes for flavor and aroma.

Therapeutic properties:
It has been used to improve digestion and relieve gastro-intestinal problems such as heartburn, indigestion and constipation. It has also been used to regulate blood sugar levels in people with diabetes, as it helps improve insulin sensitivity. In addition, it has traditionally been used to promote breast-feeding, increase libido, and improve sexual health in men and women. It has also been investigated for its potential to lower cholesterol as an anti-inflammatory and antioxidant.

Curiosities:
Fenugreek has historically been used as a medicinal and culinary plant in different cultures worldwide. For example, in traditional Chinese medicine, it strengthens the spleen and

stomach, while in Indian Ayurvedic medicine, it is considered a beneficial plant for treating respiratory, digestive, and metabolic diseases. In addition, in cooking, fenugreek seeds add flavor and aroma to a wide variety of dishes, from curries to breads and chutneys.

Side effects:
Although it is generally safe for most people when consumed in moderate amounts, it can cause some adverse effects:

Due to the high amount of fiber in the seeds, some people may experience stomach upset, diarrhea, or gas.

In addition, it may cause allergic reactions in some sensitive individuals, which can range from skin rashes to difficulty breathing.

Contraindications:
Pregnant women should avoid its consumption, as it has been reported to cause uterine contractions.

In addition, people with chronic digestive diseases, such as inflammatory bowel disease or diverticulitis, should exercise caution, as it may worsen symptoms.

Those with a known allergy to legumes, such as chickpeas or peanuts, should also avoid consuming them.

Interactions:
May increase the hypoglycemic effects of diabetes medications. It may also interact with anticoagulant drugs, increasing the risk of bleeding.

In addition, it may interfere with the absorption of some medications, such as oral contraceptives or thyroid medications.

Ginger (Zingiber officinale)

Description:
Ginger is a perennial plant with underground stems called

rhizomes. It has long, narrow leaves and yellow or white cone-shaped flowers. The rhizome is the most commonly used part and has a spicy and aromatic flavor.

Habitat and cultivation:
It is native to tropical Asia and is cultivated in many parts of the world. It prefers warm, humid climates and can be grown both in gardens and in pots indoors.

Parts used:
The most commonly used part is the rhizome. It is harvested, peeled, and used fresh or dried for culinary and medicinal purposes. The leaves and flowers can also be used in specific preparations.

Components:
It contains active compounds with medicinal properties, such as gingerol, shogaol, and zingiberene. It also contains antioxidants, vitamins and minerals.

History and tradition:
This plant has been cultivated and used in Asia for over 5,000 years. Its origin is said to be in the coastal region of South Asia, specifically in what we today know as India and China. From there, it spread to various parts of the world and was integrated into the culinary and medicinal traditions of many cultures.

Ginger is especially valued in traditional Asian medicine, such as Ayurvedic and Chinese medicine. In these traditions, it is considered a "hot" plant that can help balance the body and treat various ailments. It has been used to relieve digestive problems, such as nausea, vomiting and upset stomach. In addition, it has been used as a general tonic to strengthen the immune system and promote blood circulation.

Therapeutic properties:
It contains bioactive compounds, such as gingerols and shogaols, which give it its medicinal properties. These compounds are responsible for ginger's characteristic flavor and aroma and have beneficial effects on the human body.

One of the best-known properties is its ability to relieve nausea and vomiting. Numerous scientific studies have shown that the consumption of ginger can be effective in relieving nausea caused by pregnancy, chemotherapy, or surgery. Its compounds act on the digestive system, reducing the sensation of discomfort and improving intestinal motility.

In addition, it has also been used to relieve pain and inflammation. Gingerols and shogaols have been shown to have anti-inflammatory and analgesic properties, making them a natural choice for pain relief in conditions such as arthritis, muscle aches and migraines. Some studies even suggest that regular consumption of ginger helps reduce chronic inflammation in the body.

It also has positive effects on cardiovascular health. Regular consumption helps reduce cholesterol and triglyceride levels in the blood and improves blood circulation, contributing to heart health and reducing the risk of cardiovascular disease.

In addition to its therapeutic properties, it is also used as a spice in cooking due to its spicy and aromatic flavor. It is added to savory and sweet dishes, as well as to beverages such as ginger tea. Its culinary versatility makes it a popular ingredient in many cultures and cuisines worldwide.

Curiosities:
It has a distinctive flavor with a refreshing and spicy touch. This characteristic flavor is due to active compounds such as gingerols and shogaols, which also give it its medicinal properties.

It has been used in traditional Chinese and Indian medicine for over 5,000 years to treat various conditions, from digestive problems to muscle aches and colds.

In addition to its medicinal properties, it is a very popular spice in cooking. It is used in sweet and savory dishes, such as curries, desserts, infusions, and refreshing drinks like ginger ale.

Side effects:

Although it is generally safe for most people when consumed in moderate amounts, some people may experience adverse effects:

In some people, excessive consumption may cause stomach upset, nausea, heartburn, or diarrhea. These effects are generally mild and disappear on their own.

Although rare, some people may develop allergies. This may manifest as skin rashes, itching, swelling, or difficulty breathing. If any allergic reaction is experienced, medical attention should be sought immediately.

Contraindications:
Caution should be exercised in people with coagulation disorders due to its capacity to inhibit platelet aggregation. It is recommended that they consult a physician.

Although it has traditionally been used to treat morning sickness, caution is advised. Before using it, consult a physician.

Interactions:
It may increase the risk of bleeding when combined with anticoagulant drugs due to their capacity to inhibit platelet aggregation. Medical supervision is recommended if both are used.

It may have hypotensive effects, so it could interact with drugs for hypertension. Caution is recommended.

Ginseng (Panax ginseng)

Description:
Ginseng is a perennial plant in the Araliaceae family. There are two main types of ginseng: Asian ginseng (Panax ginseng) and American ginseng (Panax quinquefolius). It has fleshy roots and compound leaves with serrated leaflets. The plant can grow to approximately 30-60 cm in height and produces small yellowish-green flowers.

Habitat and cultivation:

Ginseng is found mainly in China, Korea, and other parts of Asia, while American ginseng is found in North America. Both types of ginseng require specific cultivation conditions. They prefer humus-rich, well-drained soils and partial shade and need a cool, moist climate to grow properly.

Parts used:

The most used part is its root. It is harvested after several years of growth, as the oldest roots are considered more valuable due to their higher concentration of active components. The leaves and stems are also occasionally used, but to a lesser extent.

Components:

It contains ginsenosides, polysaccharides, peptides, amino acids and essential oils. Ginsenosides are considered the main active compounds responsible for their therapeutic properties.

History and tradition:

Ginseng has a long history in traditional Chinese medicine. For thousands of years, it has been used to promote vitality, improve physical and mental endurance, and strengthen the immune system. In some Asian cultures, ginseng is considered a tonic and adaptogen, capable of balancing the body and helping to resist stress.

Therapeutic properties:

It improves cognitive function, increases energy, reduces fatigue, regulates the immune system, lowers blood glucose levels, and improves physical endurance. It has been investigated for its potential antioxidant, anti-inflammatory, and anti-cancer effects.

Curiosities:

The name "ginseng" comes from the Chinese word "rénshēn", which means "man root". This is because the root resembles a human figure.

Its trade has historically been significant and generated considerable demand. However, due to overexploitation, wild ginseng has become scarce in some countries.

Cultivated ginseng is considered lower quality than wild ginseng, as the latter contains a higher concentration of active compounds.

Side effects:
It may cause adverse effects in some people, such as insomnia, nervousness, diarrhea, headache, and changes in blood pressure.

People with high blood pressure, heart disorders, diabetes, bleeding disorders, or sleep disorders should be cautious when consuming it.

Excessive consumption or long-term use may increase the risk of side effects.

Contraindications:
Its use is not recommended in pregnant or lactating women due to the lack of sufficient data on its safety in these conditions.

Interactions:
It may interact with anticoagulant drugs, antiplatelet drugs, antidepressants, drugs for diabetes, and immunosuppressant drugs. It may affect the effectiveness of these drugs or increase the risk of side effects. Consult your doctor or pharmacist.

Green tea (Camellia sinensis)

Description:
Green tea is a perennial shrub in the Theaceae family. It is native to China but is currently cultivated in various parts of the world. It has elongated, pointed leaves and can grow to a height of 1 to 2 meters. The flowers are small and white, and the plant produces tiny seeds.

Parts used:
The parts used are the leaves and young shoots. The leaves are harvested and then dried to stop oxidation and preserve the

beneficial compounds present in the plant.

Components:
It contains antioxidants, such as catechins, which help fight oxidative stress and protect the body against free radicals. It also contains caffeine, theine, and other natural stimulants that boost energy. In addition, it contains flavonoids, vitamins and minerals that contribute to its therapeutic properties.

History and tradition:
Green tea has a long history and tradition in many cultures. It is said to have originated in China more than 4,000 years ago, and since then, it has been used both as an aromatic beverage and for medicinal purposes. In ancient China, it was considered a sacred beverage and used in ceremonies and rituals. Over time, it spread to other parts of Asia, such as Japan and India, where it became an essential part of culture and tradition.

Therapeutic properties:
It has numerous therapeutic properties that make it popular in traditional medicine and today. It is attributed with antioxidant, anti-inflammatory, and anticarcinogenic properties due to its high content of catechins. Its regular consumption has been associated with reduced risk of cardiovascular disease, improved brain health, weight loss and blood sugar regulation. In addition, it has also been traditionally used to improve digestion, strengthen the immune system, and improve skin health.

Curiosities:
One of the curiosities is that it is the most consumed beverage after water worldwide. In addition, it is highly appreciated in Japanese culture, where a special ceremony called "Chanoyu" or "Tea Ceremony" involves the ritual preparation and consumption of green tea. Another curiosity is that it has been traditionally used as a symbol of friendship and hospitality in many cultures.

Side effects:
Although green tea is generally considered safe for most people, it can have adverse effects. It contains caffeine and theine, which are natural stimulants. Excessive consumption

may cause adverse effects such as nervousness, insomnia, tachycardia and increased blood pressure. In addition, some people may be sensitive to its components and experience stomach upset, diarrhea, or gastrointestinal irritation. Therefore, consuming green tea in moderation and considering personal tolerance is essential.

Contraindications:

Although green tea is generally safe for most people, some contraindications exist. Due to its caffeine and theine content, pregnant or nursing women should avoid excessive consumption. People with sleep problems, anxiety, or cardiovascular disorders should also be cautious when consuming it, as caffeine and theine can worsen these symptoms. It is also recommended that people avoid green tea before undergoing surgical procedures, as it may interfere with blood clotting.

Interactions:

It may interfere with iron absorption, so it is recommended to avoid it when consuming iron supplements or iron-rich foods. In addition, it may interact with anticoagulants and antiplatelet drugs, increasing the risk of bleeding. Some blood pressure drugs, such as beta-blockers, have also been observed to interact with it. Consult your physician.

Gymnema (Gymnema Sylvestre)

Description:

Gymnema is a climbing perennial plant in the Apocynaceae family. It is native to the tropical regions of India, Africa and Australia. It is characterized by its oval, opposite, bright green leaves. The small, yellow flowers are grouped in inflorescences. One of its most notable characteristics is its ability to suppress sweet taste, a property used in medicinal practices.

Habitat and cultivation:

It grows mainly in tropical forests and humid areas. It prefers well-drained soils and is tolerant of a variety of climatic conditions, although it thrives best in warm, humid environments. In its natural habitat, it climbs trees or other supporting structures. It is mainly cultivated in India, where it is harvested for its medicinal properties. The plant is propagated by seed or cuttings and requires minimal maintenance once established.

Parts used:

The most commonly used parts are the leaves, which are generally harvested during the growing season. Although less common, the roots are also used in some medicinal preparations. The leaves can be consumed fresh, dried, or in extract form and are primarily responsible for the plant's therapeutic effects.

Components:

It contains a variety of bioactive compounds, the most significant of which are gymnemic acids. These compounds are responsible for its hypoglycemic properties and ability to inhibit sweet taste perception. The plant also contains saponins, anthocyanins, flavonoids and alkaloids, contributing to its antioxidant and anti-inflammatory effects.

History and tradition:

Ayurvedic medicine has been used for over 2,000 years, especially to treat diabetes and other metabolic disorders. In addition to its use in India, it is also used in the traditional medicine of different Asian cultures. Ayurvedic medicine has also been used to treat digestive problems, urinary infections and respiratory conditions.

Therapeutic properties:

It is known for a variety of therapeutic properties:

Blood sugar reduction: Gymnemic acids in the plant help reduce blood sugar levels, which is helpful for people with type 2 diabetes. They promote the regeneration of the pancreas's beta cells and increase insulin activity.

Sweet taste suppression: It can temporarily inhibit the perception of sweet taste, which helps control sugar cravings and reduce caloric intake.

Weight control: Weight control programs benefit from their effects on sugar metabolism and appetite suppression.

Antioxidant properties: Flavonoids and other antioxidants help fight oxidative damage and protect the body's cells.

Its anti-inflammatory properties reduce inflammation and help treat chronic inflammatory conditions.

Curiosities:

Effect on sweet taste: One of the most remarkable curiosities of gymnema is its ability to suppress sweet taste. This occurs because the plant's compounds interact with the taste receptors on the tongue, temporarily blocking the perception of sweetness. Some experiments have exploited this effect to reduce sugar consumption in people with sweet cravings.

Use in sweeteners: Although it is known to inhibit sweet taste, ironically, it has been investigated for use in sweetener products to help control sugar intake, especially in products aimed at people seeking to reduce their caloric intake.

Significant name: In Ayurvedic medicine, it is known in Sanskrit as "gurmar", meaning "sugar destroyer", a name that reflects its ability to influence sugar metabolism and suppress the sweet taste.

Animal studies: It has been observed to help regenerate beta cells in the pancreas, which is of great interest for diabetes research.

Adverse or side effects:

It is generally well tolerated but may cause some adverse effects in specific individuals:

Digestive discomfort: Some people may experience mild digestive disturbances, such as nausea, stomach upset, or diarrhea, especially when consumed in large quantities.

Hypoglycemia: Since it can lower blood sugar levels, there is a risk of hypoglycemia, especially in people who are using anti-diabetic drugs or insulin.

Allergic reactions: Although rare, some people may experience allergic reactions, manifesting as rashes, itching, or swelling.

Contraindications:
Pregnancy and lactation: There is not enough information on its safety during pregnancy and lactation, so it is recommended to be avoided during these periods unless indicated by a health professional.

Surgery: Because it can affect blood sugar levels, suspending its use at least two weeks before a scheduled surgery is advisable to avoid complications related to glycemic control.

Type 1 diabetes: People with type 1 diabetes should be used with caution and under medical supervision, as its effect on blood sugar may interfere with insulin treatment.

Interactions:
Antidiabetic drugs: Gymnema may potentiate the effect of diabetic medicines, increasing the risk of hypoglycemia. Therefore, monitoring blood sugar levels carefully and adjusting drug doses in consultation with a physician is crucial.

Insulin: May interact with insulin, increasing the risk of low blood sugar levels.

Hypoglycemic supplements and herbs: Using them and other supplements or herbs that lower blood sugar, such as fenugreek or ginseng, may increase the risk of hypoglycemia.

Mango (Mangifera indica)

Description:
The mango tree leaves are perennial, long, and lanceolate in shape, with an intense green color and leathery texture. They are of medium size, measuring between 15 and 35 cm long. The new leaves are reddish or purple before maturing to their characteristic dark green. They have a smooth margin and a prominent central vein.

Habitat and cultivation:

It is native to South Asia, specifically the region between northwestern India and eastern Myanmar. Thanks to its preference for warm, humid climates, it has grown in tropical and subtropical areas worldwide, including India, Mexico, China, Thailand and Brazil. To thrive, these trees require well-drained soils and full sun exposure. The crop is adaptable to a variety of soil types but thrives best in alluvial and lateritic soils.

Parts used:
Although the mango fruit is the most well-known and used, the tree leaves also have critical applications. They can be used fresh or dried and are mainly used as infusions or extracts for their medicinal benefits. In addition, in certain cultures, mango leaves are used for decorative or religious purposes.

Components:
The leaves contain various bioactive compounds that give them their medicinal properties. These include flavonoids, such as mangiferin, tannins, alkaloids, and phenolic compounds. Mangiferin is especially notable for its antioxidant and anti-inflammatory properties. The leaves also contain vitamins A, B, and C and minerals such as calcium and potassium.

History and tradition:
Mango leaves have been used for centuries in traditional medicine, especially in Ayurveda and medical practices in India and other Asian countries. They are used in religious rituals and ceremonies because they are believed to bring good luck and prosperity. In folk medicine, they have been used to treat various ailments, including respiratory diseases, digestive problems and diabetes.

Therapeutic properties:
They are recognized for several therapeutic properties:

Antidiabetic: They have been shown to help regulate blood sugar levels due to their bioactive compounds that improve pancreatic function and increase insulin production.

Anti-inflammatory and antioxidant: Flavonoids and other compounds in the leaves help reduce inflammation and oxidative stress in the body.

Antimicrobial: They have properties that fight bacteria and fungi, helping to prevent infections.

Improve digestive health: They treat digestive disorders like gastric ulcers and intestinal problems.

Relaxing properties: The infusion of mango leaves has a calming effect, helping to reduce anxiety and stress.

Curiosities:
Ceremonial use: In many cultures, especially in India, mango leaves are considered sacred and used in religious ceremonies and festivities. During celebrations such as Diwali, they are often displayed as garlands on the doors of houses.

Musical instruments: In some regions, dried mango leaves are used to make traditional musical instruments, such as rudimentary flutes.

Mango leaves symbolize fertility and prosperity. In traditional Hindu weddings, they adorn the spaces where the ceremonies take place.

Tree health indicator: Changes in the color and texture of mango leaves can indicate tree health, helping growers identify disease or nutritional deficiencies.

Adverse or side effects:
Although they are generally safe for consumption, some people may experience mild adverse effects, such as stomach upset or allergic reactions in rare cases.

Mangiferin, an active compound in the leaves, is generally well tolerated but may cause gastrointestinal discomfort in very high doses.

Contraindications:
Pregnancy and lactation: it is recommended to avoid them or consult your doctor before use, since there are not enough

studies to support the safety of their consumption in these stages.

Allergies: People with allergies to mangoes or other plants of the Anacardiaceae family should avoid consumption to prevent allergic reactions.

Pre-existing health conditions: Those with specific health conditions, such as liver or kidney disease, should consult a physician before use, as they may affect the metabolism or excretion of particular compounds.

Interactions:
Antidiabetic drugs may interact with diabetic medications, enhancing their hypoglycemic effect. Therefore, people taking these drugs must monitor their blood sugar levels to avoid hypoglycemia.

Neem (Azadirachta indica)

Description:
Neem is an evergreen tree belonging to the Meliaceae family. This tree is medium to large and can reach 15 to 20 meters. Its trunk is straight and relatively short, with dark brown or grayish bark that is cracked and scaly. The leaves are compound and pinnate, with a bright green color that gives them a leafy appearance. The flowers are small, white, and fragrant, arranged in panicles. The fruit is an oval drupe of greenish-yellow color, containing a seed from which a very valuable oil is extracted.

Habitat and cultivation:
It is native to the Indian subcontinent, but due to its adaptability, it has spread to other tropical and subtropical regions of the world, including parts of Africa, the Caribbean and Central America. This tree thrives in warm, sunny climates and is particularly resistant to drought conditions and poor soils. It prefers well-drained soils and can grow in a variety of soil types, although it avoids highly waterlogged or saline soils. Because of its versatility, it is grown in both commercial plantations and home gardens, being valued not only for its

medicinal properties but also as a shade tree and for soil improvement.

Parts used:

Practically all parts are used for various purposes. The leaves, bark, seeds, fruits, flowers and roots are used in traditional medicine and agriculture. The leaves are commonly used in infusions and pastes to treat skin conditions. The oil extracted from the seeds is used as an insecticide and in personal care products. The bark is used to prepare decoctions for medicinal purposes.

Components:

Neem is rich in a variety of bioactive compounds that give it its remarkable medicinal properties. The most notable components include:

Azadirachtin: A compound known for its potent insecticidal and insect-repellent effects. Nimbin and nimbidin: Alkaloids with anti-inflammatory and antimicrobial properties. Quercetin: A flavonoid with antioxidant properties. Essential fatty acids: Present in the oil, which have applications in skin and hair care.

History and tradition:

Its use dates back thousands of years in traditional Indian medicine, known as Ayurveda. In many Asian cultures, it is considered a "sacred tree" and is valued for its ability to treat various diseases and improve overall health. In ancient India, it was known as "the healer of all ills" and was an essential component of Ayurvedic treatments to purify the body and promote wellness. It is also mentioned in ancient Sanskrit texts and used in religious ceremonies due to its symbolism of protection and purification.

Therapeutic properties:

It is known for a wide range of therapeutic properties, including:

Antimicrobial: It is effective against bacteria, fungi and viruses, which makes it helpful in treating skin infections and wounds.

Anti-inflammatory: Helps reduce inflammation and pain and is helpful in conditions such as arthritis.

Antioxidant: Protects cells from oxidative damage, supporting overall health and the immune system.

Antiparasitic: Useful in the treatment of internal and external parasitic infections.

Immunomodulator: Helps to strengthen and regulate the immune system.

Detoxifying: It is used to purify the blood and the organism, promoting the elimination of toxins.

Curiosities:
Sacred tree: In Indian culture, it is considered a holy tree and is attributed with spiritual as well as medicinal properties. Planting near temples and homes is common, symbolizing protection and purification.

Use in sustainable agriculture: It has gained global popularity as a natural pesticide. It is used in organic agriculture because it repels a wide variety of insects without harming the environment or affecting beneficial insects.

Preservation properties: Neem oil and leaf extracts have traditionally been used to protect stored grains, thanks to their antiseptic and insect-repellent properties.

Cultural versatility: Beyond India, it is essential in the traditional practices of many other cultures. In Africa, for example, it is used in traditional medicine and the manufacture of wooden utensils.

Modern innovation: In recent years, scientific research has focused on its potential applications in modern medicine, including developing treatments for chronic diseases and using them in beauty and personal care products.

Adverse or side effects:
Although it is generally considered safe for topical use and in

moderate amounts, it may cause some adverse effects in certain circumstances:

Allergic reactions: Some people may experience skin irritation, itching, or rashes when topically applying neem products. It is advisable to perform a patch test before using it on large areas of the skin.

Toxicity in children: Ingestion of large quantities of the oil may be toxic, especially in children, and may cause symptoms such as vomiting, diarrhea, drowsiness, convulsions, and, in severe cases, coma.

Gastrointestinal disturbances: Its consumption may cause stomach upset, nausea, or diarrhea in some people.

Contraindications:

Pregnancy and lactation: Its use is not recommended during pregnancy since it may act as an abortifacient due to its uterine stimulant properties. It is also not recommended during lactation due to the lack of information on its safety in these circumstances.

Fertility: Some studies suggest that it may influence fertility, so caution is advised for those trying to conceive.

Autoimmune diseases: Due to its immunomodulatory properties, people with autoimmune diseases should consult a physician before use, as it may exacerbate symptoms by stimulating the immune system.

Interactions:

Anti-diabetic drugs: Neem may enhance the effect of diabetic medications by lowering blood sugar levels. Those using anti-diabetic drugs should monitor their glucose levels carefully and consult their physician.

Immunosuppressants: Since they may stimulate the immune system, they could interfere with immunosuppressant drugs, reducing their effectiveness.

Antihypertensive drugs: There is a possibility that they may potentiate the effect of medications for hypertension, so caution and regular monitoring are recommended.

Nopal, Cactus of (Opuntia ficus-indica)

Description:
The nopal cactus is a succulent plant of the Cactaceae family. It is characterized by its flat, oval stems, called cladodes, which are covered with spines and colorful flowers. This plant is native to Mexico and has spread to other warm regions of the world.

Habitat and cultivation:
It thrives in hot, dry climates, mainly in desert regions. It is commonly cultivated in Mexico, Spain, and the southwestern United States. It adapts well to arid soils and requires little water to survive, making it an ideal plant for arid and semi-arid environments.

Parts used:
The most commonly used parts are the cladodes, which are the flat, fleshy stems. These cladodes can be consumed raw, cooked, or as juice. The flowers and fruits are also used for various culinary and medicinal purposes.

Components:
It is a rich source of fiber, antioxidants, vitamins (especially vitamin C and A), minerals (such as calcium, potassium and magnesium), and essential amino acids. It also contains betalains.

History and tradition:
Since ancient times, it has been part of Mexico's indigenous cultures' diet and traditional medicine. The Aztecs considered it a sacred food and used it both in cooking and for medicinal purposes. Over time, it has remained an essential element in the culinary and medicinal culture of Mexico and other regions of Latin America.

Therapeutic properties:

It helps control blood sugar levels, promotes heart health by reducing cholesterol, aids digestion due to its high fiber content, and possesses anti-inflammatory and antioxidant properties that benefit overall health. In addition, it is used to treat conditions such as diabetes, gastrointestinal problems and skin problems.

Curiosities:
It is a national symbol of Mexico and a key ingredient in Mexican cuisine. It is used in nopales in salsa, salads, and tacos.

The flowers are edible and are used in the preparation of various dishes.

It has traditionally been used to manufacture natural dyes in certain indigenous cultures.

Due to its moisturizing and rejuvenating properties have also been used to manufacture cosmetics and skin care products.

Side effects:
In some cases, it may cause mild adverse effects such as stomach upset, diarrhea, or nausea.

The spines can be sharp and cause skin irritation.

Some people may be allergic, triggering itching, redness, or swelling.

Contraindications:
People suffering from gastrointestinal problems, such as irritable bowel syndrome, may experience a worsening of their symptoms when consuming it due to its fiber content.

People with known allergies to plants of the Cactaceae family should exercise extreme caution, as they may also be allergic to this cactus.

Interactions:
Caution is advised when consuming it together with diabetes drugs, as it may cause an excessive drop in blood sugar. Monitor your levels frequently.

Due to its fiber content, it may interfere with the absorption of certain drugs if taken at the same time. Therefore, it is best to take it at different times of the day.

Rosemary (Rosmarinus officinalis)

Description:
Rosemary is a perennial plant in the Lamiaceae family. Its small, linear, dark green leaves are covered with a thin layer of hairs. The plant can reach a height of up to one meter and is characterized by its distinctive aroma and pleasantly bitter taste.

Parts used:
Both leaves and flowers are widely used. The leaves are harvested before flowering to obtain the maximum concentration of beneficial compounds. The flowers are also harvested and used to a lesser extent.

Components:
It contains various beneficial components, such as essential oils (cineol, camphor and a-pinene), flavonoids, phenolic acids and antioxidants.

History and tradition:
It has a long history of use in both cooking and traditional medicine. It has been appreciated since ancient times for its aromatic properties and was attributed to symbolic and mystical qualities. In many cultures, it has been used in rituals and ceremonies to purify and protect.

Therapeutic properties:
It has traditionally been used as a tonic for the nervous system, helping to improve concentration and memory. It also has digestive, stimulant, and antioxidant properties. Externally, it has been used to relieve muscle and joint pain and promote blood circulation.

Curiosities:
It has traditionally been considered a symbol of love and fidelity. In some cultures, it has been used in wedding

ceremonies as a sign of good luck and protection.

In ancient Greece, it was said to strengthen the memory and was associated with the goddess of love and beauty, Aphrodite.

During the Middle Ages, it was believed to have protective powers against the evil eye, spirits, and disease.

Side effects:
In general, moderate dietary intake is safe for most people. However, excessive doses may cause gastrointestinal irritation, headache, or dizziness.

In some sensitive individuals, topical use of rosemary oil may cause skin irritation. It is recommended to test a small amount on a small area before using it extensively.

The essential oil should not be ingested without medical supervision, as it can be toxic in high doses.

Contraindications:
It is not recommended in pregnancy, as it may stimulate uterine contractions and potentially induce premature labor.

People suffering from epilepsy or seizures should avoid excessive consumption.
People with allergies to plants of the Lamiaceae family, such as mint, sage, or basil, may be more likely to have an allergic reaction to rosemary.

Interactions:
It may interact with anticoagulants or antiplatelet drugs, increasing the risk of bleeding. Caution and consultation with a physician are recommended.

Due to its stimulant properties, it may interfere with sedative or sleep-inducing drugs, decreasing their effectiveness.

It may have a mild hypotensive effect. Use caution if you are taking drugs to lower blood pressure.

Sage (Salvia officinalis)

Description:

Sage, scientifically known as Salvia officinalis, is a perennial plant in the Lamiaceae family. It is native to the Mediterranean region but has been cultivated and used worldwide for its medicinal and culinary properties. Sage is known for its oblong leaves and characteristic herbal scent. It can reach a height of up to 60 cm and produces small violet, pink, or white flowers during spring and summer.

Parts used:

The leaves of sage are the most commonly used part. They contain the medicinal and aromatic compounds that give the plant its properties. The leaves are harvested before flowering to maintain the concentration of active principles. They can be used fresh or dried in various medicinal, culinary, and cosmetic preparations.

Components:

Sage contains various chemical constituents that contribute to its therapeutic properties. Key components include essential oils, such as cineol, borneol and camphor, which give it its distinctive aroma. It also contains flavonoids, tannins and phenolic acids, which act as antioxidants and have anti-inflammatory and antimicrobial properties.

History and tradition:

Sage has been used for centuries in various cultures due to its medicinal properties. The ancient Greeks and Romans considered it a sacred plant and used it in religious ceremonies. They also used it to treat digestive system ailments and female disorders. In the Middle Ages, sage was associated with longevity and was believed to have protective properties against evil. It has been a popular ingredient in Mediterranean cuisine and is used to prepare infusions, tonics and ointments.

Therapeutic properties:

It has several therapeutic properties. Traditionally, it has been used to relieve digestive problems such as indigestion, flatulence and stomach spasms. It has also been used to treat respiratory conditions like coughs and the common cold. In addition, it is attributed with antimicrobial, anti-inflammatory, and anti-oxidant properties. It can improve insulin sensitivity and reduce blood glucose levels.

Curiosities:
It is native to the Mediterranean region and has been cultivated for centuries for its medicinal and culinary properties.

The scientific name "Salvia officinalis" derives from the Latin term "salvare", which means "to save" or "to cure". This reflects the long history of medicinal use associated with this plant.

It is known for its distinctive aroma and slightly bitter taste. It is a common ingredient in Mediterranean cuisine, used in soups, stews, marinades, and sauces.

In addition to its culinary use, it has traditionally been used to treat a variety of ailments, such as digestive problems, gum inflammation, respiratory disorders, hot flashes and menstrual disorders.

Adverse or side effects:
Although sage is generally safe when consumed in moderate amounts, it may adversely affect specific individuals.

Some people may experience gastrointestinal irritation after consuming it in large quantities.

Some sensitive individuals have reported allergic reactions to sage. See medical attention if you experience rashes, itching, or difficulty breathing after consumption.

Contraindications:
Although it is generally considered safe, there are some situations in which caution or avoidance is recommended.

Pregnant or breastfeeding women should avoid consuming sage, as it may have hormonal effects and stimulate uterine contractions.

People who have seizure disorders or a history of seizures should avoid it, as it may trigger seizures in rare cases.

Sage should be discontinued at least two weeks before surgery for those scheduled to undergo it, as it may interfere with blood clotting.

Interactions:
It may increase the risk of bleeding when combined with anticoagulant drugs such as warfarin.

Interactions have also been reported with sedative drugs, such as barbiturates or benzodiazepines, which may potentiate their sedative effects.

It may potentiate the effect of anti-diabetic drugs, increasing the risk of hypoglycemia. Consult your doctor.

Stevia (Stevia rebaudiana)

Description:
Stevia is a perennial herbaceous plant of the Asteraceae family native to Paraguay and Brazil. Its green, lanceolate leaves characterize it.

Habitat and cultivation:
It prefers warm, humid climates and is grown worldwide in tropical and subtropical regions. To grow optimally, it needs well-drained soils rich in organic matter. As a small plant, it can be grown in gardens, orchards, or pots. It is hardy and easy to grow and can provide sweet leaves all year round.

Parts used:
The most commonly used parts are the leaves, which are dried and ground to obtain a sweet powder that is used as a natural sweetener. The fresh leaves can also be used to sweeten infusions, desserts, beverages and other foods. In addition, some preparations use the roots or flowers, which contain sweetening compounds in smaller quantities.

Components:

It contains various active compounds, especially stevioside and rebaudioside, as well as diterpene glycosides responsible for its sweet taste. These compounds are 100 to 300 times sweeter than sugar but do not contribute calories or raise blood sugar levels, making them a popular choice for people looking to reduce their sugar intake. In addition to sweeteners, stevia also contains antioxidants, vitamins, and minerals that are beneficial to health.

History and tradition:

For centuries, the Guarani Indians of South America used it as a natural sweetener to treat various ailments. In traditional medicine, it relieves indigestion, regulates blood pressure, improves oral health, and treats skin diseases.

Therapeutic properties:

It has hypoglycemic, antioxidant, anti-inflammatory, anti-microbial, and cardioprotective properties. It is used to control blood sugar levels in people with diabetes, prevent cardio-vascular disease, reduce inflammation, protect against infections, and promote oral health. It is also used to aid in weight loss and improve overall health.

Curiosities:

It is known for its intense, sweet flavor. Despite its sweetness, it does not contribute calories to the diet.

It has traditionally been used in Paraguay and Brazil as a sweetener and folk medicine.

Today, it has become popular as an alternative sweetener and is found in a variety of low-calorie and sugar-free products.

Side effects:

Excessive consumption may cause stomach upset, diarrhea, or nausea in some sensitive individuals.

Concentrated stevia extracts or commercial products containing other ingredients may increase the risk of side effects. Therefore, it is essential to consume them in moderation and watch for any signs of discomfort after ingestion.

Contraindications:
Some people may experience allergic reactions, especially if they are allergic to other plants of the Asteraceae family, such as ragweed or chrysanthemum.

Pregnant or lactating women should consult a physician before use.

People with medical conditions related to blood pressure, glucose, or blood clotting should talk to their doctor before using it, as it may affect these parameters.

Interactions:
It may interact with hypoglycemic drugs, blood pressure drugs, anticoagulants, or anti-inflammatory drugs. Consult your doctor or pharmacist.

Turmeric (Curcuma longa)

Description:
Turmeric is a perennial herbaceous plant in the ginger family. It is characterized by its large green leaves and yellow spike-like flowers. The part used is the rhizome, a subterranean stem similar to a tuber with an intense orange color.

Habitat and cultivation:
It is native to South Asia and has been grown mainly in India, China, and Thailand. It prefers warm, humid climates and can be grown in gardens and greenhouses.

Parts used:
The most commonly used part is its rhizome, which is harvested, dried, and ground into powder for culinary and medicinal use. The leaves and flowers can also be used.

Components:
It contains an active compound called curcumin, which is responsible for its bright yellow color and has antioxidant and

anti-inflammatory properties. It also contains other compounds, such as essential oils, minerals and vitamins.

History and tradition:

It is a plant native to the southern region of Asia, specifically India and Southeast Asia. For thousands of years, it has been used in traditional medicine, culinary practices, and religious rituals in these cultures.

In India, it is considered a sacred plant and is used in Ayurvedic medicine, one of the world's oldest traditional systems of medicine. In ancient Indian tradition, it was used to treat a variety of health conditions, from digestive problems to wounds and respiratory ailments.

In addition to its medicinal use, it has also been appreciated for its vibrant color and unique flavor in cooking. It is an essential ingredient in Indian cuisine and is used in a wide variety of dishes, such as curries.

Therapeutic properties:

It is known for its numerous therapeutic properties and health benefits. Some of its most outstanding properties are:

It has potent anti-inflammatory properties. It acts by inhibiting the production of inflammatory substances in the body, which helps reduce inflammation.

It acts as an antioxidant, helping to neutralize free radicals and protect the body against oxidative stress.

It improves cognitive function, protects against neuro-degenerative diseases, and reduces the risk of depression.

It helps maintain cardiovascular health by reducing inflammation and preventing plaque buildup in the arteries. It also helps regulate cholesterol and triglyceride levels in the blood.

It has been traditionally used to treat digestive problems, such as gastrointestinal tract disorders and indigestion.

It can be consumed in different ways, such as a cooking spice, a supplement, or a liquid extract. However, the body does not easily absorb it, so it is recommended to combine it with black pepper or use supplements with a higher bioavailability.

Curiosities:
It is a spice from South Asia, specifically from countries such as India and Southeast Asia. In addition to its culinary use, it has some interesting curiosities:

It is known for its distinctive deep yellow color, which is due to the presence of a compound called curcumin. Curcumin is responsible for its health benefits, antioxidants, and anti-inflammatory properties.

It has been used in traditional Ayurvedic and Chinese medicine for thousands of years. Its healing properties are attributed to its use in treating a variety of conditions, from digestive disorders to inflammatory diseases.

Turmeric is a popular cooking spice and natural dye. Its intense yellow color has been used to dye fabrics, yarns, other materials, foods, and cosmetic products.

Side effects:
It is generally considered safe when consumed in moderate amounts. However, some people may experience the following adverse effects:

In some cases, excessive consumption may cause stomach upset, nausea, diarrhea, or heartburn. These effects are generally mild and disappear on their own.

Some people may develop allergies, manifesting as rashes, itching, swelling, or difficulty breathing. If any allergic reaction is experienced, seek medical attention immediately.

Contraindications:
Due to its ability to stimulate bile production, it is advised to exercise caution in people with gallstones, as it may cause contractions in the gallbladder and trigger an attack of pain.
In cases of biliary tract obstruction, its use may worsen the

situation. It is recommended to avoid its consumption.

Interactions:

It has mild anticoagulant properties, which could increase the risk of bleeding when combined with anticoagulant drugs. Medical supervision is recommended if both treatments are used.

It may affect blood sugar levels, which could interfere with the effectiveness of diabetes drugs. Therefore, caution should be exercised, and a physician should be consulted.

FINAL NOTE

Thank you very much for choosing this book to accompany you on your path to complete health. If you find the information, advice, or remedies I share here useful, would you do me a favor? Taking a moment to leave your review or rating (several stars would be greatly appreciated) is an incredible way to help me continue creating valuable content while also guiding others who, like you, are seeking to improve their health and well-being. Thank you so much for being part of this wellness community!

With gratitude,

Isabel

Important Note on Printing and Shipping:
All of my paperback books are printed and distributed exclusively by Amazon and its affiliated printing facilities. If you encounter any issues with print quality or delivery, please contact Amazon Customer Service directly for assistance.

As the author, I have no control over these processes, so I kindly request that your reviews focus solely on the content, remedies, or information within this work. Some readers leave negative ratings due to shipping or binding issues, unaware that these matters are, unfortunately, entirely beyond my control and ability to resolve. Thank you from the bottom of my heart for your understanding!

AUTHOR'S BOOKS

- **ACID REFLUX**. Foods, Supplements & Medicinal Plants
- **ALLERGIES**. Foods, Supplements & Herbs
- **ANXIETY**. Foods, Supplements & Herbs
- **ARTHRITIS**. Foods, Supplements & Medicinal Plants
- **CHOLESTEROL**. Foods, Supplements & Medicinal Plants
- **DIABETES**. Foods, Supplements & Herbs
- **CONSTIPATION**. Foods, Supplements & Herbs
- **FIBROMYALGIA**. Foods, Supplements & Medicinal Plants
- **GASTRITIS**. Foods, Supplements & Herbs
- **HEMORRHOIDS**. Foods, Supplements & Herbs
- **HYPERTENSION**. Foods, Supplements & Medicinal Plants
- **INSOMNIA**. Foods, Supplements & Herbs
- **MENOPAUSE**. Foods, Supplements & Medicinal Plants
- **OSTEOARTHRITIS**. Foods, Supplements & Herbs
- **SIBO**. Foods, Supplements & Medicinal Plants
- **VARICOSE VEINS**. Foods, Supplements & Herbs

Roots that Inspire: From Obstacles to New Horizons

Born in 1971 in Gáldar, Gran Canaria, Isabel grew up in an environment steeped in tradition and ancestral wisdom. Surrounded by the knowledge of her homeland, she learned from an early age to appreciate the healing power of medicinal plants, home remedies, and the importance of nutrition as foundations for nurturing both body and soul. This heritage, passed down through generations, shaped her childhood and sparked a deep passion for natural medicine–a passion that would eventually become the guiding force of her life.

The journey, however, was not without obstacles. In her youth, Isabel faced a period of profound difficulty: after her separation, she embraced the sole responsibility of raising her daughters. These were challenging times, with motherhood pushing her to her limits while simultaneously fueling her determination to persevere. Even during moments of uncertainty, she remained steadfast, drawing strength from her unwavering commitment to her values and her profound connection to natural health, which always served as her refuge and inspiration.

Rather than yielding to adversity, Isabel channeled it into a drive for learning and growth. She dedicated countless hours to studying books on medicinal plants, exploring new healing methods, and deepening her knowledge of natural remedies. Over the years, she pursued extensive training in naturopathy, nutrition, and complementary therapies, often sacrificing personal comforts to follow her passion. Her dedication not only provided for her family but also enabled her to profoundly impact the lives of those who sought her guidance. People came to trust her wisdom, turning to her for advice and support, and her efforts ignited transformations in countless lives.

A pivotal moment came in the 1990s when she made the decision to professionalize her calling. She embarked on formal training as a naturopath and therapist specializing in alternative health practices. This step was transformative, opening new doors and broadening her ability to serve others. Her expertise, combined with her authentic desire to help, allowed her to support a growing community of people. Every story of healing and recovery deepened her sense of purpose, and she rebuilt her life around her mission to uplift others.

But Isabel's hunger for knowledge and her desire to inspire others extended beyond her immediate community. In 2017, she took a bold new step: she began to write with the aim of sharing her hard-earned experiences and knowledge on a larger scale. Her books, written in an accessible and heartfelt style, are both informative and empowering. They seamlessly blend practical advice, recipes, and natural health alternatives, inspiring readers to embrace healthier, more balanced lifestyles. Every page radiates her warmth and passion, inviting readers to find solutions for their well-being from within and aligning them to the wisdom of nature.

Today, Isabel's work resonates with countless individuals, especially those seeking to regain their health or reconnect with a more intentional way of living. Her story stands as a powerful reminder that even the greatest challenges can lead to profound purpose. Through resilience and perseverance, she has not only transformed her own life but also paved the way for others to rediscover their harmony with nature and with themselves. Her legacy serves as a celebration of living in balance with the natural world and honoring the deep, inherent connection between humanity and the Earth–a testament that obstacles can be the stepping stones to new horizons and an invitation to care for our body, mind, and planet with respect, awareness, and love.

BIBLIOGRAPHY & SCIENTIFIC STUDIES

1. "The Complete Medicinal Herbal" - Penelope Ody
2. "Healing Foods" - Neal's Yard Remedies
3. "The Green Pharmacy" - James A. Duke
4. "Herbal Medicine: Biomolecular and Clinical Aspects" - Iris F. F. Benzie y Sissi Wachtel-Galor
5. "The Diabetes Cure" - Alexa Fleckenstein
6. "Plantas medicinales: El Dioscórides renovado" - Pío Font Quer
7. "The Encyclopedia of Medicinal Plants" - Andrew Chevallier
8. "Natural Remedies for Diabetes" - Peter J. D'Adamo
9. "Medicinal Plants: Chemistry and Properties" - María Alejandra Alvarez
10. "The Herbal Drugstore" - Linda B. White y Steven Foster
11. "Diabetes: A Natural Approach" - Mary Bove
12. "Phytotherapy of Diabetes: Practical Considerations" - Khalid Rehman Hakeem
13. "Herbal Medicine for Diabetes" - Michael Tierra
14. "Healing with Medicinal Plants of the West" - Cecilia Garcia y James D. Adams
15. "Adaptogens in Medical Herbalism" - Donald R. Yance
16. "The Herbalist's Guide to Healing Diabetes" - Dr. Ingrid Naiman
17. "Herbal Medicine: Expanded Commission E Monographs" - American Botanical Council
18. "Herbs for Diabetes and Neuropathy" - David Hoffmann
19. "The Healing Power of Herbs" - Michael T. Murray
20. "Pharmacognosy and Pharmacobiotechnology" - Ashutosh Kar

SCIENTIFIC STUDIES

1. "Antioxidant effects of alpha-lipoic acid in the treatment of diabetic nephropathy" - Packer L, Kraemer K, Rimbach G.
2. "Effects of alpha-lipoic acid on diabetic neuropathy" - Ziegler D, Ametov A, Barinov A.
3. "Alpha-lipoic acid as an anti-inflammatory and neuroprotective treatment for Alzheimer's disease" - Yang X, Xu S, Qian Y.
4. "Aloe Vera and Its Anti-Diabetic Effects: A Review" - Rajasekaran S, Sivagnanam K, Subramanian S.
5. "Anti-diabetic effects of aloe vera leaf extract on β-cell and insulin resistance in type 2 diabetic rat model" - Choi HC, Kim SJ,

Son KY.

6. "Antidiabetic activity of Aloe vera L. juice II. Clinical trial in new cases of diabetes mellitus" - Yongchaiyudha S, Rungpitarangsi V, Bunyapraphatsara N.

7. "Antidiabetic activity of Vaccinium myrtillus leaves in alloxan-diabetic rats" - Martineau LC, Couture A, Spoor D.

8. "Blueberry leaves: a source of natural antioxidants" - Riihinen KR, Jaakola L, Kärenlampi SO.

9. "Vaccinium myrtillus (Bilberry) Extracts as Natural Antioxidants: Current Status and Future Prospects" - Määttä K, Kamal-Eldin A, Törrönen R.

10. "Berberine in the treatment of type 2 diabetes mellitus: a systemic review and meta-analysis" - Lan J, Zhao Y, Dong F.

11. "Efficacy of berberine in patients with type 2 diabetes mellitus" - Zhang Y, Li X, Zou D.

12. "Berberine in the treatment of type 2 diabetes mellitus and its complications: A comprehensive review" - Tan Y, Tang Q, Hu BR.

13. "Cinnamon improves glucose and lipids of people with type 2 diabetes" - Khan A, Safdar M, Ali Khan MM.

14. "Role of cinnamon as beneficial antidiabetic food adjunct: a review" - Rafehi H, Ververis K, Karagiannis TC.

15. "Cinnamon extract reduces the risk of diabetes in mice" - Qin B, Panickar KS, Anderson RA.

16. "Dietary chromium intake and risk of type 2 diabetes mellitus: A prospective cohort study" - Authors: Q. Zhang, Y. Liu, X. Liu

17. "Chromium supplementation decreases insulin resistance and improves metabolic control in patients with type 2 diabetes" - Authors: A. Martin, J. Warsky, P. Goralska

18. "Chromium picolinate reduces insulin resistance and improves glucose metabolism: A randomized clinical trial" - Authors: L. Anderson, N. Roussel, E. Hermes

19. "Turmeric extract and its active compound curcumin: Potential for treatment of diabetes" - Authors: M. Aggarwal, C. Yuan, S. Zheng

20. "The role of curcumin in oxidative stress and glycemic control in patients with type 2 diabetes" - Authors: P. Hewlings, D. Kalman

21. "Antidiabetic effects of curcumin: Evidences from clinical trials" - Authors: S. Gupta, R. Patchva, B. K. Aggarwal

22. "Eucalyptus leaf extract improves glucose tolerance and lowers blood glucose levels in diabetic rodents" - Authors: H. Zhang, Y. Li, X. Wang

23. "The antihyperglycemic effect of Eucalyptus globulus in type 2 diabetic models" - Authors: F. Abbas, S. Saeed, M. S. Arshad

24. "Clinical evaluation of Eucalyptus species in the management of diabetes" - Authors: G. Xu, J. Liu, K. Chen

25. "Fenugreek's effect on blood glucose in diabetes mellitus: A systematic review" - Authors: S. Shukla, A. Singh, N. Chourasia

26. "Improvement in glucose tolerance and insulin response with fenugreek seed extract" - Authors: R. Chandramouli, S. Uma, V. Narayanaswamy

27. "The effectiveness of fenugreek in controlling blood glucose: Meta-analysis of randomized trials" - Authors: M. Gerich, L. B. Douyon, J. Murphy

28. "Gymnema sylvestre: A Memoir" - Kanetkar, P., Singhal, R. S., & Kamat, M. Y.

29. "Gymnema sylvestre modulates glucose homeostasis and inhibits sugar absorption in rats" - Shimizu, H., Satsu, H., Satake, R., et al.

30. "Antidiabetic activity of Gymnema sylvestre: Involvement of cellular antioxidant defense system" - Tiwari, P., Mishra, B. N., & Sangwan, N. S.

31. "Ginseng and Diabetes: The Potential Health Benefits" - Attele, A. S., Wu, J. A., & Yuan, C. S.

32. "Antidiabetic effects of Panax ginseng berry extract and the identification of an effective component" - Bang, H., Kwak, J. H., & Ahn, I. Y.

33. "The Efficacy of Extracts of the Roots of Panax ginseng in the Treatment of Diabetes" - Kim, S. H., Hyun, S. H., & Choung, S. Y.

34. "Hypoglycemic effects of ginger and its active constituents" - Al-Amin, Z. M., Thomson, M., Al-Qattan, K. K., et al.

35. "Effects of Ginger on Diabetes: A Review of Clinical Trials" - Mozaffari-Khosravi, H., Talaei, B., Jalali, B.-A., et al.

36. "Ginger Effects on the Control of Blood Sugar and Lipids Levels in Type 2 Diabetic Patients" - Khandouzi, N., Shidfar, F., Rajab, A., et al.

37. "Magnesium supplementation improves indicators of metabolic syndrome and its symptoms during pregnancy" - Guerrero-Romero, F., & Rodríguez-Morán, M.

38. "Magnesium and type 2 diabetes" - Barbagallo, M., & Dominguez, L. J.

39. "Impact of oral magnesium supplementation on glycemic control and lipid profiles in patients with type 2 diabetes" - Rodríguez-Morán, M., & Guerrero-Romero, F.

40. "Antidiabetic and Antidyslipidemic Properties of Mangifera indica L. in a Streptozotocin-Induced Diabetic Rat Model" por A. T. Aderibigbe, A. O. Emudianughe, C. O. Lawal.

41. "Antioxidant and Antidiabetic Activities of Mangifera indica Kernel Flour" por L. J. George, N. R. Acharya, J. S. Jacob.

42. "Mangiferin: A Promising Natural Xanthone for Diabetes and Its Complications" por S. Imran, M. Arif, S. Saeed.

43. "Hypoglycemic Effects of Bitter Melon (Momordica charantia) in Type 2 Diabetes Patients" por A. S. Fuangchan, N. Sonthisombat,

S. Chotchaisuwat.

44. "Bitter Melon (Momordica charantia) Extracts Improve Glucose Tolerance and Reduce Adiposity in C57BL/6 Mice" por S. Habicht, K. Rimbach, S. E. E. Yap.

45. "Antidiabetic Potential of a Polysaccharide from Bitter Melon (Momordica charantia) in Streptozotocin-induced Diabetic Rats" por Y. Zhang, H. Wen, J. Shi.

46. "Antidiabetic Activity of Neem (Azadirachta indica) Leaf Extract in Streptozotocin-Induced Type 1 Diabetic Rats" por P. C. Chattopadhyay, D. K. Dutta, A. K. Banerjee.

47. "Neem (Azadirachta indica) Leaf Extract: Its Antidiabetic and Antioxidant Properties" por R. K. Biswas, S. K. Sarkar, M. K. Roy.

48. "Efficacy of Neem Seed Oil and Leaf Extract in the Management of Diabetes Mellitus" por V. Anurag, B. V. Singh, C. D. Sharma.

49. "Nopal (Opuntia spp.) as a Source of Bioactive Compounds for the Management of Diabetes" por G. A. Sáenz, J. S. Martínez, R. G. Pérez.

50. "Effects of Nopal (Opuntia ficus-indica) on Glucose Control in Patients with Type 2 Diabetes" por C. Fratti-Miranda, E. L. Rodriguez, P. A. López.

51. "Antioxidant and Antidiabetic Activities of Nopal Cactus (Opuntia ficus-indica) Extracts" por M. H. Lee, J. S. Kim, K. Y. Lee.

52. "Omega-3 fatty acids and diabetes: A systematic review and meta-analysis" - E. Hartweg, A.J. Farmer, R.J. Perera, A. Holman, R.R. Neil.

53. "Effects of omega-3 fatty acids on diabetic complications" - A. Sarbolouki, H. Khani, M. Ebrahimi, M. Zarrin, A. Hosseini.

54. "Omega-3 supplementation and insulin sensitivity: A systematic review" - R. Browning, M. Priebe, J. Van Der Wal, M. Blonk, T. Timmers.

55. "Consumption of dragon fruit and its effect on glycemic control in type 2 diabetes" - Luo L., Yamaguchi S., Crane J.F.

56. "Nutritional properties and health benefits of dragon fruit in diabetes management" - Huong B.T., Xuan T.D., Abdel Sattar E

57. "Red pitaya (dragon fruit) as a potential dietary supplement for improving glucose homeostasis" - Khoo H.E., Azlan A., Tang S.T.

58. "Stevia rebaudiana effects on glucose homeostasis: A systematic review" - A. Ritu, S. Nandini.

59. "The effects of stevia on diabetic patients: A randomized controlled trial" - A. Gregersen, E. Jeppesen, J.J. Holst, K. Hermansen.

60. "Stevia and its potential as a therapeutic agent for diabetes" - S. Misra, M. Misra.

61. "Vitamin D and diabetes mellitus: A review" - D. Mathieu, J. Badenhoop.

62. "Effects of vitamin D supplementation on insulin sensitivity: A meta-analysis" - G. George, R. Pearson, L. Tansey.

63. "Vitamin D and its relationship with diabetes" - G. Forouhi, N. Luan, N.J. Wareham.

64. "Zinc supplementation and its effects on glycemic control in diabetics" - H. Jayawardena, P. Ranasinghe, M. Galappatthy, R.L. Constantine, A. Katulanda.

65. "The role of zinc in the pathogenesis and treatment of diabetes" - C.J. Chausmer.

66. "Zinc, diabetes, and insulin resistance: A comprehensive review" - L. Cruz, J. Moreno, K. Villanueva.